STOP TREADING WATER AND DROWN
Plummeting to a Spirit-led Life

Sophia Christie

STOP

Treading Water and Drown

Plummeting to a Spirit-led Life

Your Light Publishing

Requests and comments should be directed to:
Your Light Publishing
P. O. Box 1067
New Market VA 22844
yourlight@zoho.com

Printed in the United States of America.
FIRST EDITION

Contents

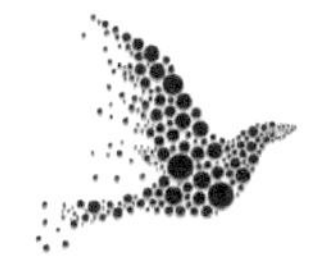

This book is dedicated to all the lonely, the sick and the lost – and to those who have tried and failed and yet whose heart is pure.

FOREWORD

I am a blessed mom. I am amazed at the awesomeness of God. His thoughts and ways are not anticipated, not understood. How can a daughter who has undergone abandonment and pain continue to rise above day after day?

My daughter told me she was writing a book. She always shared scripture with me, but I was not prepared for the chapters that started to arrive in the mail. I cried when I read some of the details of her life that I was not aware of. I felt chills when I read what was obviously divinely inspired. I smiled at the chapter titles. Through this book, my daughter was teaching me what surrender to the Creator meant. Not that I could learn that in one book reading, but it opened my eyes to see the daily miracles in my own life and ways to gain strength and courage. If I'm having a bad day or am feeling overwhelmed, I can pick up her book on the table next to where I have my morning coffee, and read a few paragraphs or lines of scripture.

We live in an angry world. We argue about how to fix it. We demand changes in laws, more security. The last thing anyone wants to hear is surrender, "let go." Step outside on a clear night, look at the stars and envision the vastness of the universe. Don't you wish you could tap into the wisdom that created all of that? You can. This book will give you an in-road into how to start that journey to wisdom and peace of mind, not from a scholar, but from a young woman who has struggled, been broken, and restored.

Grace and peace!

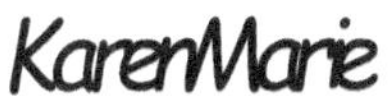

A NOTE FROM THE AUTHOR...

I sat there in shock as I read the line on the piece of paper in front of me, "Reason for admittance: homicidal/suicidal thoughts." All my life I tried to be a good person, giving people the benefit of the doubt, being a good friend. I was the type of person who rooted for the underdog and would give the shirt off her back if she could. Yet during the 10 days I was in the hospital, no one came to visit me, to hold my hand, or to give me a hug. The culmination of my life had come to this point: sitting in the Emotional Recovery Center at Virginia Beach Psychiatric Center, wondering *How in the world did I end up here?* At the time, my four children were all under the age of twelve. My life's efforts had been in vain. I had found no fulfillment in life, no inner peace, no answers as to why I was even alive. I was more lost than ever.

I believe that we all have big questions. Why am I here? What's this life for? Why is there so much suffering? I was In my twenties, and my life was not turning out as I had hoped.

Growing up, I had very supportive parents. I took ballet and gymnastics. I learned to play the flute and was a drum major in high school. I even took four years of Latin because I wanted to be a doctor. My mom and dad were always there to encourage and support me. Our family went to church every Sunday and took vacations together. I always had my own room, had chores to do and rules to follow, and earned an allowance. My mother was a stay-at-home mom and was "mom" to many of my friends in the neighborhood. My dad taught me to change a tire before learning to drive and matched me dollar for dollar on my first car. My parents had been married for twenty-five years before he passed away. My mother still lives in the first house they bought and has had the same phone number for over forty years. I figured that my life would turn out the same way. Little did I know that the stability I had known throughout my life was the envy of many people. Years passed before I realized what a blessing my childhood really was.

When I became pregnant out of wedlock at nineteen, my dreams of traveling the world were shattered. In search of hope, I turned to the Catholic church. The priest told me to recite some Hail Marys and seemed to present the sense that everything would be okay. I didn't buy it. My son's father wasn't exactly supportive; he was in love with someone else. He wanted to do the right thing, but it never really worked out that way. Shortly after my son was born, my father died suddenly. He was only 48 years old. I had no answers as to why these things were happening, and life was not making sense to me at all. So, I became angry: angry with my family, angry with myself, angry with God.

My anger had turned to despair.

At first, I tried joining the world in its vanity and pleasure-seeking schemes. I sought money and validation, so I became an exotic dancer. Spending time in all the wrong places and doing all the wrong things only drove me further into darkness. I married my son's father out of obligation but began dabbling in drugs and alcohol. I was frequently abused by my husband, and I hadn't spoken to my mother for quite some time. By the time I became pregnant with my daughter, I found myself living in a homeless shelter for women and children. It was there that I seriously began to seek the truth. I knew I needed something that the world could not offer. My anger had turned to despair. During that dark time, I began to see God in a whole new way. I made amends with my mother and started earnestly praying and studying the Bible. I thought for sure I would find answers to all my questions. I even went as far as becoming a Jehovah's Witness. I tried moving away and making it on my own, to no avail. I reunited with my children's father only to be disappointed again. I felt unloved and worthless. And I was now pregnant with twin boys.

In utero, the smaller of the two was diagnosed with a severe heart condition that required surgery almost immediately after birth. He was born with CHARGE syndrome, which entailed seeing numerous specialists and having multiple surgeries. The first few years of his life were filled with hospital stays, therapy, and at one point he was home on oxygen and a feeding tube. The circumstances kept his father and I together, for a time. My son's condition eventually stabilized but the relationship I had with his father never did. One night during an explosive episode, I realized that one of us would literally "have to go." That is how I ended up at the Psychiatric Center.

The hospital sent me back home on anti-depressants and ordered me to go to counseling. That, too, was short-lived. I stayed with my mother for a short time. But ultimately, I ended up packing just a few bags and my twin boys, who were now four years old, into a used minivan that my mother bought for me, and driving several hundred miles away from home, in hopes of starting over yet again. My eldest son and daughter were gone with their father—to where I didn't even know. I fell back on religion and began attending church and reading the Bible again. Though the custody battle was raging, life seemed to be rather peaceful. However, it didn't last. The children's father ended up in a psychiatric unit himself, and as a result, my two older children came to live with me as well. I spent several years in and out of court, never getting to any real conclusion. I was frustrated with the system, with religion, and with life. Everything seemed so out of control, and I was struggling in every area of my life. My children's father never paid child support, went to jail for a year, and blamed me for everything that went wrong. My kids resented me, the Jehovah's Witnesses disfellowshipped me, and I felt as if the walls around me were caving in. Still, I was left with no answers to my questions.

The definition of insanity is repeating a particular action over and over expecting a different result. I can honestly say that I have been there. Even our culture is insane. It convinces us that the more we do and the more we accomplish, the better we are. So, I aimed to just keep trying harder. But because my focus was wrong, all my efforts only wore me out. I worked long and hard, never getting ahead. I began to see myself as insignificant and felt that my life was pointless. My ability to logically consider anything had vanished, and I was making extremely poor decisions. I was depressed and angry. Instead of facing the truth and trials of my life head-on, I began to find ways of escaping them. Then I hit what some would call "rock bottom." I lost my home. I lost my kids. I lost "me" or, at least, who I thought was "me." All my efforts, once again, had been in vain. Not only was I still lost, but now I was also very much alone.

There is no greater invitation to live than the diagnosis of death.

Blaming others got me nowhere. Accepting responsibility made me feel guilty, but, ironically, the guilt kept me from doing anything. I continued focusing on what *was* while neglecting what could be. I had to experience pitfalls and some serious mistakes before I learned to embrace the pain of regret. Avoiding it only led to more confusion. "No pain, no gain," as the famous boxer, Muhammad Ali, would say. Just as a doctor would, I had to examine my pain to get to the root of my problem. Only then could I get clarity. I knew that the pain was there to get my attention, but I didn't know what to do about it.

There is no greater invitation to live than the diagnosis of death. It is unfortunate that it takes a death sentence for some of us to want to live better. I believe it is because we misbelieve. We procrastinate, thinking that there is always tomorrow. Time, however, is a temporary gift and no one really knows how many moments he or she will get to experience in this life. If we truly understood that, we would spend our time more wisely. I have come to believe that life is not a goal to be achieved but rather a gift to be received. As I journey through my life, I treasure each moment and am grateful to enjoy every opportunity that comes my way. I believe what the Quakers teach: Everyone possesses his own gifted form, referred to as inner light, which is "that of God." Our Creator wants us to know who we really are and why we are here. Before we get so busy telling our lives what to do, we should stop and listen.

I am convinced that God is greater than any difficulty.

Doing the right thing is not the most comfortable thing to do. In fact, it is often the most uncomfortable thing. Repentance is one of those uncomfortable things. Call it what you will, an enlightenment, an awakening, a reckoning. All those things are the politically-correct way of life telling you that you've got it all wrong, and it's time for a change. In this book, I simply want to share with you the perspective that changed my way of life. It didn't make all my problems go away, nor did it answer all my questions. However, learning to walk by Spirit and not by sight has been the single most impactful lesson of my life. I am, by no means, an expert, and I continue to grow each day. But the peace that surpasses understanding is mine, and the ability to accept my reality without distress is a precious gift. Although unlearning the ways of the world is challenging, I am convinced that God is greater than any difficulty. My prayer is that you will not only gain some insight from the pages that follow but that you will ultimately come to love your Creator—and the life He has given to you—even more.

Peacefully yours,

Sophia Christie

APPRECIATIONS

First and foremost, my Heavenly Father Jehovah, whose loving devotion to me is timeless and whose Amazing Grace is truly AMAZING!

Jesus Christ, my redeemer and friend, whose kindness and mercy is endless and whose love has made this book possible.

My faithful husband, who has patiently supported me and inspired me to be all who God created me to be. I am deeply grateful for your music, your voice and your love.

My mother, who has loved me with her tender heart, and whose words will always be a source of encouragement. It has been a treasure to share this project with you.

My family and friends, whose presence in my heart, decorate my life. You add meaning to my world and I love each one of you.

My editor, Angela Ivey, whose expertise, proficiency and direction was right on time.

Thank you all!

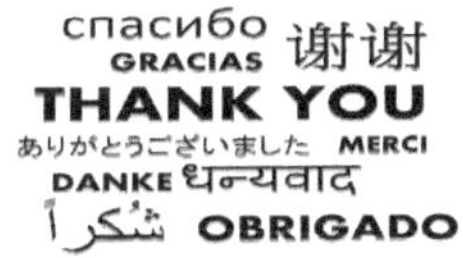

Chapter 1

PLAYING POSSUM

"You can do it!" "Keep it up!" "Try again!" It was not uncommon to hear those words from my teachers, coaches or my parents. Growing up with such support taught me to keep trying even when things were difficult. However, I found that using the same prescription as an adult only led me to exhaustion. I spent years thinking that, if I kept trying, kept going, I would make it to somewhere better than where I was. I was *wrong*. In fact, my life was deteriorating. Before I was even forty years old, I had become a struggling, single mom of four, working 60 plus hours a week at a job that barely paid the bills. *My* marriage had failed, and I was alone. *My* kids weren't happy, and I didn't have time for them. *My* family was far away, and I felt abandoned. *My* friends were few, if any. *My* thoughts were not good, and *my* outlook was bleak. *My* life seemed to have developed its own momentum and I was out of control. I knew I was failing miserably at my life, but the only thing I knew to do was to just keep going. There was a thirst in my life that could not be quenched, and eventually, I lost all that I had been struggling to keep. I was left dazed, confused, and angry.

---

*Inevitably, poor inner work leads to
poor outer work.*

In a commencement speech, Denzel Washington once said, "Remember just because you are doing a lot more doesn't mean you're getting a lot more done. Don't confuse movement with progress."[1] If our "keep on keeping on" is only occupying time and we aren't progressing, we are simply wasting our energy and attention. We can be so convinced that we are *doing* all the right things that we neglect to see that our *thinking* is off-course. Inevitably, poor inner work leads to poor outer work.

I remember clearly the moment it happened. I was overwhelmed with grief and desperation. I deeply wished that I could feel glad to be alive, but my emotional pain was so severe that I honestly wanted my life to just be over. I found myself sitting in my car one night, sobbing. I *gave up*. I let go of everything—all that I had, all that I wanted, all that I thought I knew. I could not go on like I had been, so I handed myself over, torn and empty, to God. I remember complete silence, and then...a glimmer of hope. I could almost feel God's unseen hands holding me, like a newborn baby in his mother's arms. I knew then that God's promise to never forsake me was real. Isaiah 49:16 tells us, "See, I have engraved you on the palms of my hands; your walls are ever before me" and I saw that in this very moment. It was as if God commanded the storm within me to be still, and it obeyed. I then believed there was hope—a *calm amidst the chaos*. In the apostle Paul's letter to the Corinthians, he says, "Our bodies are made of clay, yet we have the treasure of the Good News in them. This shows that the superior power of this treasure belongs to God and doesn't come from us. In every way we're troubled, but we aren't crushed by our troubles. We're frustrated, but we don't give up. We're persecuted, but we're not abandoned. We're captured, but we're not killed. " (2 Corinthians 4:7-9 GWT). I knew in that moment that I was not alone.

When we find ourselves in a difficult situation, our inclination is to find a way out. However, what we do while trying to escape can sometimes lead to our demise. For example, when a person is suffering from severe hypothermia, he will often disrobe. *This makes absolutely no sense.* Removing your clothes in extreme cold only causes rapid heat loss, which speeds up the process of freezing to death. Although science has termed this "paradoxical undressing," no one seems to have the answer as to *why* humans do this. Proverbs reminds us that "There is a way which seems right to a man, but its end is the way of death" (Proverbs 14:12 BSB). Even when we aren't facing eminent death, however, we may say and do things that contradict our very goals. The apostle Paul said it this way, "I don't really understand myself, for I want to do what is right, but I don't do it. Instead, I do what I hate" (Romans 7:15 NLT). No one is immune to making mistakes or wrong turns, but it is what we do when we find ourselves in those places that makes all the difference in the end. We can choose to ignore our mistakes and repeat them or admit them and learn from them. The key is to realize that we often need help in doing so.

It is simply not possible to be a person of integrity without thinking matters through before we act. Benjamin Franklin said, "If you fail to plan, you are planning to fail." In other words, unintentional living is risky business. Even Jesus said, "Which of you, wishing to build a tower, does not first sit down and count the cost to see if he has the resources to complete it? Otherwise, if he lays the foundation and is unable to finish the work, everyone who sees it will ridicule him, saying, 'This man could not finish what he started to build.'" (Luke 14:28-30 BSB). Yet, even in thinking things through, our view is still limited and making plans based on a lack of correct information will only give rise to failure. All it takes is to look at our world to see this simple fact. Even with the best of structural engineering, we can still build bridges and dams that fail. Marriages fail amongst even the most dedicated Christians. Seemingly healthy individuals can possess hearts and kidneys that fail. That is why I say that there is danger in a self-willed life. The old saying that *what you don't know can't hurt you* is simply not true. Jeremiah 10:23 echoes this idea: "Lord, I know that people's lives are not their own; it is not for them to direct their steps."

Even our own opinions and life experience can cloud our ability to see our life's purpose. Take, for instance, the Ugly Duckling. He didn't know who he was. He tried following the crowd in order to fit in and listening to everyone he met. He ended up being misinformed, mistreated, and rejected. The lesson of the story at the end is best summed up by Hans Christian Andersen:

It bent its head down upon the water, expecting nothing but death. But what was this that it saw in the clear water? It beheld its own image; and, lo! it was no longer a clumsy dark-gray bird, ugly and hateful to look at, but a—swan! It matters nothing if one is born in a duck-yard if one has only lain in a swan's egg. It felt quite glad at all the need and misfortune it had suffered, now it realized its happiness in all the splendor that surrounded it.[2]

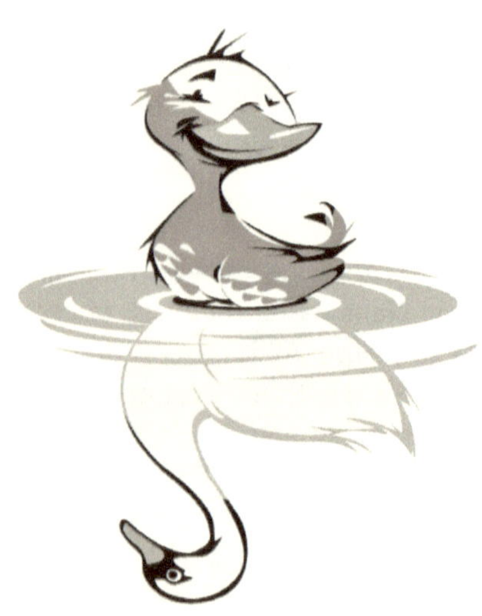

We, too, must realize that circumstance does not make us who we are and that our purpose was determined prior to our production. Just like the ugly duckling whose true identity was there all along, so is ours. We only need to discover it. Doing so while finding joy in our troubles and happiness in our reality can often be quite challenging on our own. Indeed, "With man this is impossible, but with God all things are possible" (Matthew 19:26).

The founder of Bahamas Faith Ministries International, Myles Munroe, once said, "Not knowing the purpose of a thing inevitably leads to abuse of a thing."[3] The next obvious thing to ask then is how do we come to know our purpose? There's a scene in the Disney movie *The Little Mermaid*[4] in which Ariel finds a fork at the bottom of the ocean. She takes her treasure to her "wise" friend, the seagull. He explains to her that the fork is called a "dinglehopper" and that humans use it to style their hair. Ariel, having limited knowledge of human life, is delighted to hear it and believes it as truth. We also, in our search for answers, can be fooled by society's instructions on how we are *supposed* to live and what we are *supposed* to do. That is why it would behoove us to question those ideas and make seeking our Creator's thoughts a priority.

Life originates with and is sustained by God. He is what I would call a "life specialist." When my car needs work, I take it to my mechanic. But if my pet gets sick, my mechanic probably won't be much help. The right expert is essential to the outcome of any situation. Only God can be the most trusted adviser on how to live. Although vastly diverse in creation, each one of us is individually and uniquely designed. Our true purpose lies only in the mind of our maker.

Psalm 139 reminds us that God alone created our inner being and that every day of our life has been recorded before even one of them has taken place. God has a grand plan for this life and possesses the power to resurrect life as well: "For I know the plans I have for you," declares the Lord, "plans to prosper you and not to harm you, plans to give you hope and a future" (Jeremiah 29:11). In order to sincerely seek God, however, we must first realize that we need Him. Unfortunately, waiting to endure a personal tragedy in order to understand that we indeed need Him is the real tragedy.

You have searched me, Lord,
and you know me.
You know when I sit and when I rise;
you perceive my thoughts from afar.
You discern my going out and my lying
down; you are familiar with all my ways.
Psalm 139: 1-3

Behavioral economics teaches that a greater assortment of choices only creates a greater distance between your choice and what makes you happy. That means that the less choices you have, the closer you are to choosing something that will actually make you happy. With the plethora of competing choices that the world can offer, it is no wonder that there are so many unhappy people in it. However, in surrendering to God, there are only two choices. We either continue living for ourselves or we decide that God's way is best. Chances are, if we are at the point of choosing between those two, we already realize that living self-willed is no good for us. So, choosing God's plan is sort of a no-brainer.

Hearing the word "surrender" often conjures up charming images of an arm raised in the air, gently waving a little white flag. However, true surrender is so much more. It really means to relinquish possession of control and to give that control to another power, to cease resisting and yield. It means to stop fighting and accept defeat. But there is another verb which better describes what we should do when it comes to surrendering all to God: *acquiesce*. It comes from the Latin word for "rest" and means to accept, agree, and allow while being silent and not protesting, or to comply quietly. This reminds me of the possum, with its propensity to play "dead" when confronted by an enemy or a situation that it just doesn't know how to deal with. However, God is not our enemy and life goes on with or without us. Like the possum, we must be willing to not only lay down our lives, but to do it without an argument.

Choosing God's plan is sort of a no-brainer.

Jesus said, "I can guarantee this truth: A single grain of wheat doesn't produce anything unless it is planted in the ground and dies. If it dies, it will produce a lot of grain. Those who love their lives will destroy them, and those who hate their lives in this world will guard them for everlasting life" (John 12:24-25 GWT). He was revealing to us that *real living* is hidden within dying and that even in the greatest loss, there is greater gain. Deuteronomy 15:10 exhorts us to, "Give generously to him, and do not let your heart be grieved when you do so. And because of this the LORD your God will bless you in all your work and in everything to which you put your hand."(BSB) Tremendous reward follows those who submit to God. The master of the universe has all things at His disposal, possesses endless potential and desires much more for us than we can even fathom. That is what Paul means when he says, "No eye has seen, no ear has heard, and no mind has imagined what God has prepared for those who love him" (1 Corinthians 2:9 NLT).

However, the decision to surrender is only the first step of the journey. It is the single most pivotal moment that changed the course of my life. "You don't choose a life...you live one" is one my favorite lines from the movie, *The Way* (2010). The point here is that we can sometimes be so worried about preserving our own lives that we miss out on actually *living*. If we want to save our lives, we cannot cling to them; we must spend them. Jesus said, "Whoever wants to be my disciple must deny themselves and take up their cross and follow me. For whoever wants to save their life will lose it, but whoever loses their life for me will find it" (Matthew 16:24-25). However, sacrificing our own way of living and accepting all that a surrendered lifestyle entails is difficult. Jesus understood that well, but He showed us that successfully surrendering to His Father is possible: "For to this you were called, because Christ suffered for you, leaving you an example, that you should follow in his footsteps" (1 Peter 2:21 BSB).

Having a model to follow is certainly helpful but leaving pride behind in order to do so is a task. There is an inner struggle between our minds and our flesh that rages in most of us. What we want to do, we find ourselves not doing and vice versa. Joni Eareckson Tada[5], a now best-selling author, was paralyzed from the neck down following a diving accident when she was a teenager. She describes first realizing her condition by saying that she knew in her mind exactly what she wanted to do, but that her body was totally unresponsive. Though most of us can only relate to a small portion of the struggle she must have faced, the underlying reality of frustration is the same. Paul referred to himself as a wretched man when describing his fight but also said, "I batter my body and bring it into servitude..."(1 Corinthians 9:27 BLB). That indicates the depth and severity of the internal struggle.

If you have ever taken on a remodeling project yourself, you probably realize that having the right tool for the job is essential. Therefore, taking on a supernatural endeavor requires God's supernatural power. We must realize that we are surrendering to the kingdom of heaven, God's throne. From it flows great power and mercy. It is from that place of *grace* where infinite blessings arise. Dying to self and dedicating our lives to the One who created it removes the power of sin over us and elevates us to a position in God's favor. His promise to us is the same as it was to the apostle Paul: "My *grace* is sufficient for you, for my power is made perfect in weakness" (2 Corinthians 12:9).

God desires only our willingness to give control of our lives to Him. He already has everything taken care of for us. It is only under the shield of God's *grace* that I live and breathe, and it's amazing to see His creative energy in all I do. I received a completely new life from the inside out. Through Him, we are made knew.

And no one puts new wine into old wineskins. For the wine would burst the wineskins, and the wine and the skins would both be lost. New wine calls for new wineskins.
Mark 2:22 NLT

There is also great peace in giving over control. The fighting is over and there are no more "voices" telling you what to do, no more "forces" playing tug-o-war with you. It is so much easier to hear His voice without the struggle that confusion brings. Surrendering all also means having nothing left to hold us back or weigh us down. The residue of our previous life is washed away, making way for new beliefs and ideas to take root. Philippians 4:13 teaches that we can do all things *through* Christ. Realizing that affords me opportunities for growth in every area of my life, all because of Jesus, who is the Way, the Truth and the Life (John 14:6). Realizing His love for me has moved me from darkness into light and from lies into truth. I believe, as Paul did, that "...Christ's love compels us, because we are convinced that one died for all, and therefore all died. And he died for all, that those who live should no longer live for themselves but for him who died for them and was raised again" (2 Corinthians 5:14-15). By faith I have come to say, "It is no longer I who live but Christ" (Galatians 2:20 NLT), and I pray that you may come to say the same.

Just like an old home that has been completely restored, we can know tremendous improvement in living for God versus living for ourselves. Alexander Pope, an 18th century English poet, once wrote, "The greatest discovery of a man's heart is to see it how God sees it."[6] I have found that God's revelation of me is greater than any breakthrough I could possibly have on my own. The apostle Paul said, "To live is Christ, to die is gain" (Philippians 1:21). I now understand what he meant.

Chapter 2

DITCH THE FLOATIES

If you have ever taken swimming lessons, you probably learned how to tread water. It is intended to be a temporary help until a rescuer can reach you. Treading water expends a lot of energy and you would soon tire trying to stay above water. If you were to find yourself shipwrecked out in open water, treading water would not save your life. A better course of action would be to cling to the first floating thing you could find. That would be a wise choice. This is not the case in life. The things we often cling to actually *keep* us from our destiny. We spend too much of our energy just "treading water," hoping that someone or something will come by and rescue us. Though it may seem to be unconventional advice, I say that we need to stop "treading water" and just "drown." The drowning I speak of is the complete surrendering to God, who is our refuge and strength, a help always near in times of great trouble (Psalm 46:1). But in order to completely surrender, there are some things we absolutely need to let go of—or avoid altogether.

FEAR

Some years ago, I wanted to learn how to scuba dive. Before I could enroll, the school required me to experience what it feels like to be underwater with all the gear. So, I suited up, jumped in the pool, and went under. Breathing underwater, while being held down by weights, was disturbing for me. I stayed under for about ten minutes, but could never get comfortable. My nerves got the best of me. Once back on dry ground, I realized that scuba diving was not for me! My discomfort and uneasiness prevented me from signing up.

Most of the time, fear is an unpleasant emotion that we experience when we believe that someone or something is dangerous and/or likely to cause us pain or loss. But going through life always trying to avoid loss will never lead us to maturity. Risk is a part of life, and often, the greater the risk, the greater the reward. We hold improper beliefs that cause us to fear needlessly, or we see fear as an obstacle instead of using it as a stepping stone to victory. Persistent fear leads to worry and doubt, which keeps us listening to lies, prevents us from taking any action, and wastes valuable time. I've heard it said that worry is like a down payment on a problem that you may never have. The truth is that we don't know what tomorrow holds and wanting complete control of our circumstances and surroundings is based solely on fear. What we need to understand is that "control" is merely an illusion. King Solomon stated it this way: "I have seen something else under the sun: The race is not to the swift or the battle to the strong, nor does food come to the wise or wealth to the brilliant or favor to the learned; but time and chance happen to them all." (Ecclesiastes 9:11). There are just some things that only God can explain. Learning to embrace the loss, the pain, and the unknown is essential to casting fear aside.

Food for thought:

Have I not commanded you? Be strong and courageous. Do not be afraid; do not be discouraged, for the LORD your God will be with you wherever you go.
Joshua 1:9

So do not fear, for I am with you; do not be dismayed, for I am your God. I will strengthen you and help you; I will uphold you with my righteous right hand.
Isaiah 41:10

When you pass through the waters, I will be with you; and when you pass through the rivers, they will not sweep over you. When you walk through the fire, you will not be burned; the flames will not set you ablaze.
Isaiah 43:2

I sought the Lord and he answered me, He delivered me from all my fears.
Psalm 34:4

For the Spirit God gave us does not make us timid, but gives us power, love and self-discipline.
2 Timothy 1:7

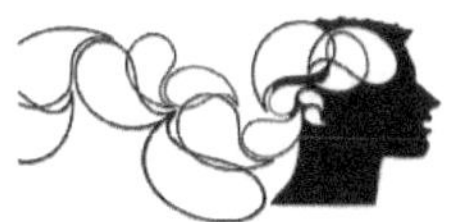

PRIDE

When I was younger, I thought I could handle anything on my own. I didn't feel like I was proud, yet saying that I didn't need anybody's help was, in fact my pride speaking. I have had to learn the hard way that, when the going gets tough, sometimes we need to ask for help. It is far better to have back-up if you need it than to need it and not have it. You may hear the same old advice from the same old people, but it is far more beneficial to be told something you've heard before than to have never heard it at all. To think you have "heard it all" is prideful. Pride is a feeling of deep pleasure or satisfaction, often stemming from one's own achievements. No matter how worthy our own accomplishments may seem, unbridled pride can cause us to be egotistical and overconfident. Therefore, we must be cautious with it. It can prevent us from listening to truth and keep us from learning from anyone or anything.

The mere ability or opportunity to do a particular thing does not always make it the right thing.

The mere ability or opportunity to do a particular thing does not always make it the right thing. Because we are limited in wisdom, we must learn to get out of our own way. When we think we "know it all," it will inevitably cause us to fall. Consider Ramses, the Pharaoh of Egypt. He was stubborn and refused to do anything other than what he wanted to do. After seeing the miraculous plagues of God, "still, Pharaoh's heart was hardened, and he did not listen to them, just as the LORD had said"(Exodus 7:13 BSB). Through his rebellion, he lost his only child, his people, his army, and his life.

No man holds greater power than God Almighty.

Pride can also cause us to make mistakes and lead us to rebel. In the Old Testament, King Nebuchadnezzar sought to be so praised that it cost him all his wealth and much more. Daniel tells him, "You will be driven away from people and will live with the wild animals; you will eat grass like the ox and be drenched with the dew of heaven. Seven times will pass by for you until you acknowledge that the Most High is sovereign over all kingdoms on earth and gives them to anyone he wishes."(Daniel 4:25). Even Nebuchadnezzar's own son, Belshazzar, lost the entire Babylonian kingdom, as well as his very life due to his arrogance. The prophet Daniel revealed to him:

> *"You have set yourself up against the Lord of heaven…you did not honor the God who holds in his hand your life and all your ways"*
> *(Daniel 5:23).*

No man is the giver and sustainer of his own life, only God is.

The book of Revelation speaks about two classes of people: the sheep and goats. Goats tend to be strong-minded and not very good followers. Conversely, sheep are easy to train and come to the voice of their shepherd. What goats fail to do, sheep naturally do. Learn to be a sheep.

Food for thought:

When pride comes, then comes disgrace,
but with humility comes wisdom.
Proverbs 11:2

Pride goes before destruction,
a haughty spirit before a fall.
Proverbs 16:18

Do you see a person wise in their own
eyes? There is more hope for a fool than
for them.
Proverbs 26:12

In his pride the wicked man does not seek
him: in all his thoughts there is no room
for God.
Psalm 10:4

For by the grace given me I say to every
one of you: Do not think of yourself more
highly than you ought, but rather think of
yourself with sober judgment, in
accordance with the faith God has
distributed to each of you.
Romans 12:3

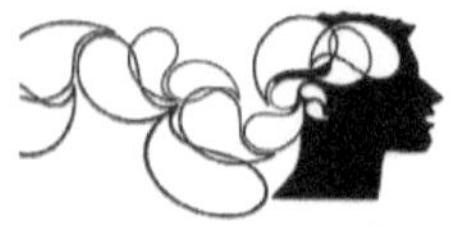

GUILT

Guilt implies fault. After we have done something wrong, even if by accident, long-term guilt, ironically, can keep us from making things right. It is debilitating. We must admit our mistakes and do our best to make amends. Acknowledging our own failure should lead us to repentance—a change in our thinking and behavior. However, when we dwell on our failures and neglect to see the hope in front of us, it can be a heavy burden to bear. In Revelation, Satan is called the "accuser of the brethren." His role as prosecutor is to pursue a guilty verdict, but we have been assigned a defense attorney—Jesus Christ—who has acquitted us: "He saved us, not on the basis of deeds which we have done in righteousness, but according to His mercy…"(Titus 3:5 NASB). We have been declared innocent through the blood of Christ's sacrifice. Learn to embrace your innocence.

Accepting a guilty verdict after you have been found innocent is to deny the grace and mercy of God.

After King David's adultery with Bathsheba, he wrote Psalm 51. David recognizes his guilt but gives it to God for cleansing. He acknowledges that his broken spirit is a pleasing sacrifice to God, and that only God's power can make his broken bones dance. However, there is a difference between guilt and regret. Often, we can make mistakes even with the best of intentions. In those cases, once we realize that our actions did not quite line up with reality, we feel regret. Both proper guilt and regret should lead us to humble ourselves before God and accept His mercy. The apostle Paul told the Corinthians:

Yet now I am happy, not because you were made sorry, but because your sorrow led you to repentance. For you became sorrowful as God intended and so were not harmed in any way by us. Godly sorrow brings repentance that leads to salvation and leaves no regret, but worldly sorrow brings death. See what this godly sorrow has produced in you: what earnestness, what eagerness to clear yourselves, what indignation, what alarm, what longing, what concern, what readiness to see justice done. At every point you have proved yourselves to be innocent in this matter. (2 Corinthians 7:9-11)

The sorrow of which Paul writes leads us to change our minds and hearts, which is acceptable to God. If we are to understand God's mercy, we in turn, must accept His forgiveness. Only God can take away our guilt and regret caused by human sin. Alexander Pope explains this simply: "To err is human. To forgive, Divine."[1]

Food for thought:

*'Come now, let us settle the matter,' says the
LORD. 'Though your sins are like scarlet, they
shall be as white as snow; though they are
red as crimson, they shall be like wool.'
Isaiah 1:18*

*I have swept away your offenses like a
cloud, your sins like the morning mist.
Return to me, for I have redeemed you.
Isaiah 44:22*

*If you, O LORD, kept a record of sins, O
Lord, who could stand? But with you there
is forgiveness.
Psalm 130:3-4*

*For I will forgive their wickedness and will
remember their sins no more.
Hebrews 8:12*

*If we confess our sins, He is faithful and
just to forgive us our sins and to purify us
from all unrighteousness.
1 John 1:9*

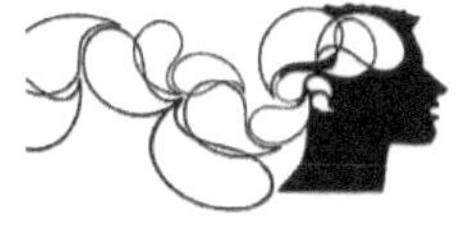

ANGER

Anger is a complex emotion. It can involve fits of rage, vengeance-seeking, resentment, animosity, or hatred towards someone or something. It can also be as simple as being irritated or annoyed by another person. On the one hand, we read about God's anger towards sin and unrighteousness and are instructed to hate what God hates. On the other, we are admonished to love even our enemies and to be slow to anger. For the sake of simplicity, let's focus on the type of anger which is harmful. There is no denying that anger exists within the human heart, but it is how we respond to it that makes the difference. As Scripture indicates, it is not what goes into a man that defiles him, but what comes out (Matthew 15:11).

When we react in rage, we risk losing loved ones and as well as our own direction in life.

The world seems to be filled with anger these days. But hatred in the hearts of men has existed since the very first family. Cain was angry that God had favored Abel's gift over his. "Why are you so angry?" the Lord asked Cain. "Why do you look so dejected? You will be accepted if you do what is right. But if you refuse to do what is right, then watch out! Sin is crouching at the door, eager to control you. But you must subdue it and be its master" (Genesis 4:6-7 NLT). Despite this warning, Cain's temper caused him to murder his own brother, and he became a wanderer for the remainder of his days. When we react in rage, we risk losing loved ones as well as our own direction in life.

In the book of Esther, Haman paid the ultimate price for his inappropriate anger. He was so enraged by the fact that Mordecai would not bow down to him, that he plotted to have him publicly hung on a pole to die. But when the truth was revealed, it was Haman himself who ended up hanging on the pole. One of King David's sons, Absalom, also harbored anger and wanted revenge. His own half-brother, Amnon, had raped his sister. So, Absalom wanted to execute punishment upon him. David loved his son Amnon, so did not demand reproach from him. Absalom was angry with his own father and grew to resent him. He decided to take matters into his own hands and lured Amnon to his death. He spent the rest of his life plotting to overthrow his father's kingdom. One day, when Absalom was out riding his mule, it ran under a tree and a branch hit Absalom in the head, killing him. Benjamin Franklin once said, "Whatever is begun in anger, ends in shame." That was certainly the case for both Haman and Absalom.

We all have been slighted or hurt by someone at least once; that's just a part of this life. Holding a grudge only leads to more want. We cannot force a person to make amends any more that we can undo what has been done. Unresolved anger will only lead to bitterness, clouded judgment, and ulcers. It is to our benefit that we learn to *let it go*.

*An angry person stirs up conflict, and a
hot-tempered person commits many sins.
Proverbs 29:22*

*Do not be quickly provoked in your spirit, for
anger resides in the lap of fools.
Ecclesiastes 7:9*

*In your anger do not sin : Do not let the
sun go down while you are still angry, and
do not give the devil a foothold.
Ephesians 4:26-27*

*My dear brothers and sisters, take note of
this: Everyone should be quick to listen,
slow to speak and slow to become angry,
because human anger does not produce
the righteousness that God desires.
James 1:19-20*

*Whoever claims to love God yet hates a
brother or sister is a liar. For whoever does
not love their brother and sister, whom
they have seen, cannot love God, whom
they have not seen.
1 John 4:20*

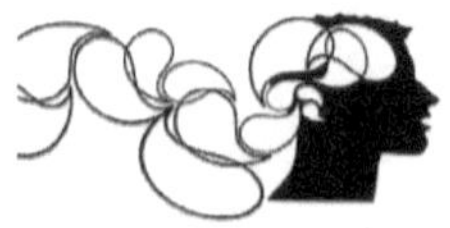

LIES

Lies emerge from countless places: media, religion, politics, culture, history, tradition, family, our minds—even our own lips. Each time the infamous character, Pinocchio, would tell a lie, his nose would grow. Although he eventually learned to tell the truth, the classic tale of Pinocchio reveals more about truth than you may think. Pinocchio earnestly wanted to become a real boy but had difficulty deciphering between the truth and lies. He was outsmarted by lying characters such as *Honest John*[2], with his sales pitch of the easy road to success. The world in which we live in is much the same—full of deception. We are all trying to find our way in this life, but it can be challenging to know what is truth and what is mere fiction. Like Pinocchio, without truth we can never reach our full potential.

Society has imposed this "fake it till you make it" mentality upon us, but faking it accomplishes nothing good. It only overrides our own need to be who we truly are and ultimately leads us to a point of failure. God holds all truth, but sometimes that truth can be hard to swallow. I used to believe that if things didn't end up like I wanted them, I was somehow suffering injustice. That was a lie. Things won't always go our way. Nor should they. Understanding that truth has given me a mindset that reduces my emotional reaction to any given circumstance. The truth, as ugly as it may seem to us, is better than any lie.

Believing a lie and telling a lie can be equally damaging. Samson was so smitten by Delilah that he believed her questions about how and why he was so strong to be innocent inquiries. In reality, his enemies had paid her money to find out and tell them, she lied and betrayed him. He lost his hair and, accordingly, his strength. In the New Testament, Ananias and his wife, Sapphira, sold a piece of property and conspired to lie about how much they had sold it for. They brought only a portion of the money to the congregation as an offering and lied directly to Peter. Peter asked, "Ananias, how is it that Satan has so filled your heart that you have lied to the Holy Spirit and have kept for yourself some of the money you received for the land?" (Acts 5:3). They were struck dead before the congregation. Both Ananias and his wife died because they attempted to cheat God and lie.

> ### *Speaking the truth and trusting the truth of God's word is a protection for us, both physically and spiritually.*

Satan is called the father of all lies. Adam and Eve had been warned by God that eating the fruit from the tree of the knowledge of good and evil would lead to their death. But the serpent lied, saying "You will not certainly die...for God knows that in the day you eat of it...you will be like God"(Genesis 3:4-5). Eve was convinced to eat the forbidden fruit, and from that day on, man has been dying—proving Satan to be the liar he really is. Both speaking the truth and trusting the truth of God's word is a protection for us, physically and spiritually.

Even flattery is a form of falsehood and can be just as damaging. Proverbs 29:5 says that "Those who flatter their neighbors are spreading nets for their feet." The classic Aesop Fable of *The Crow and The Fox* shows this lesson well.

> One day a fox once saw a crow fly off with a piece of cheese in its beak and settle on a branch of a tree. "That cheese is for me," thought the fox, as he slyly walked up to the foot of the tree.
>
> "Good-day, Miss Crow," he cried. "How beautiful you look today: how glossy your feathers are, how your eyes twinkle. I bet your voice must be

sweeter than any other bird. Oh...if I could just hear one song from you that I may greet you as the Queen of Birds."

Feeling like a queen, the crow proudly raised her head and began to caw her best, but the moment she opened her beak the piece of cheese fell to the ground, only to be snapped up by the sly fox.

We should never trust flatterers, for they live at the expense of anyone who may listen. Vice versa, it is never a good idea to boost someone's ego, especially for the sake of personal favor. Regardless of whom may be on the receiving end, flattery only seeks to compromise truth and is something to be wisely avoided. Paul cautions us against believing flatterers: "For such people are false apostles, deceitful workers, masquerading as apostles of Christ. And no wonder, for Satan himself masquerades as an angel of light" (2 Corinthians 11:13-14). In this case, flattery can get you nowhere. Fast.

Food for thought:

*The LORD detests lying lips, but he delights
in people who are trustworthy.
Proverbs 12:22*

*Do not merely listen to the word, and so
deceive yourselves. Do what it says.
James 1:22*

*Then you will know the truth, and the truth
will set you free.
John 8:32*

*Let no one deceive you with empty words,
for because of such things God's wrath
comes on those who are disobedient.
Ephesians 5:6*

*Dear friends, do not believe every spirit, but
test the spirits to see whether they are from
God, because many false prophets have gone
out into the world.
1 John 4:1*

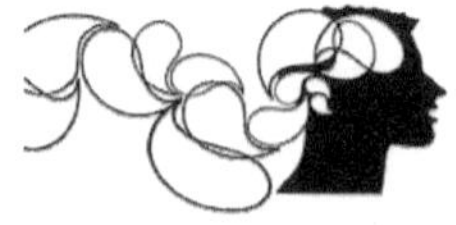

DISTRACTIONS

The modern world we are accustomed to is a far cry from the simple life. Today's world says, "the faster the better," "hurry up and get it done," "no time to wait." In addition, the world will always offer competing alternatives for your attention. We have meals to prepare, bills to pay, places to go, and people to see. A new research study performed by Microsoft[3] has confirmed that the average adult's attention span is now just eight seconds—less than that of a goldfish. The amount of time we can stay focused has been consistently decreasing as technology increases. We are being trained to multi-task in every aspect of our lives, while reducing our efficiency at any given one of them. Just as doing more does not mean we are getting more done, focusing on more does not mean we are more focused. When a camera's lens is not properly focused, the resulting photograph is blurry. We too, produce things of lesser quality when we are not attentive. Maintaining focus can be difficult, but it is possible with the right approach.

We are being trained to multi-task in every aspect of our lives, while reducing our efficiency at any given one of them.

One legendary major league baseball story illustrates this point. Hank Aaron was a famous power hitter with the Milwaukee Braves, while Yogi Berra was a well-known catcher with the New York Yankees. As their teams played against each other in the World Series, Aaron came up to bat. Yogi kept up his usual ceaseless chatter, intended to distract him. Yogi said, "Hank, you're holding the bat wrong. You're supposed to hold it so you can read the trademark." Aaron didn't say a thing. But when the next pitch came, he drove the ball hard into the left-field bleachers, smashing a home run. Upon reaching home plate Aaron looked at Yogi and said, "I didn't come up here to read."[4] That is an important lesson for us on the value of focusing. Aaron did not allow himself to be distracted by the opposition. We too, must have our minds set on God before the challenges of life come, if we want to succeed.

There is an old Jewish blessing that says, "May you always be covered by the dust of your Rabbi." Disciples never wanted to lose sight of their Rabbi. In fact, they were taught to maintain such a closeness with him that they would absorb his daily habits and mindset. It prevented them from being preoccupied with their own life and kept them focused on learning from him. Similarly, maintaining an intimate relationship with God helps to keep us focused on spiritual things. But it requires resolve and learning to ignore that which obstructs our view of God. Both of which are skills we need to cultivate. Besides, distractions will only prevent us from experiencing the blessings God has in store for us.

Food for thought:

*Be very strong; be careful to obey all that is
written in the Book of the Law of Moses,
without turning aside to the right or to the left.
Joshua 23:6*

*My son, pay attention to my wisdom, turn
your ear to my words of insight.
Proverbs 5:1*

*No one can serve two masters. Either you
will hate the one and love the other, or you
will be devoted to the one and despise the
other. You cannot serve both God and money.
Matthew 6:24*

*But when you ask, you must believe and
not doubt, because the one who doubts is
like a wave of the sea, blown and tossed
by the wind. That person should not
expect to receive anything from the Lord.
Such a person is double-minded and
unstable in all they do.
James 1:6-8*

*Therefore, dear friends, since you have been
forewarned, be on your guard so that you may
not be carried away by the error of the lawless
and fall from your secure position.
2 Peter 3:17*

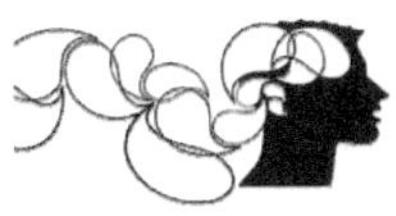

APATHY

"I don't care." Arguably three of the most dangerous words in the English language. But, also very common. Gyalwang Karmapa, a leader of the school for Tibetan monks, said, "A lack of love can cause people to have no help when they need help, no friends when they need a friend. So, in a sense, the most dangerous thing in the world is apathy. We think of weapons, violence, warfare, disease as terrible dangers, and indeed they are, but we can take measures to avoid them. But once our apathy takes hold of us, we can no longer avoid it."[5] The world tends to promote the desensitization of people. The more chaos we see, the less affected we are by it. Every school shooting seems to be less and less surprising. When we become insensitive, we do less to combat the problems we face as a people.

The same can be true regarding our own lives. So many of us are surrounded by difficulties that it can be challenging to view them as anything other than common. You can always tell what a person is passionate about by the way they speak or the things they do. Many people today, however, have no passion. They find themselves just getting by, immune to what's going on around them, unmotivated. Pink Floyd speaks of this feeling of man as being "comfortably numb."[6] Unfortunately, that way of life is both dangerous and contagious. Regardless of why a person may feel that way, complacency leads to a miserable and lonely existence. One who lives in such a way has lost hope. Without hope, one finds it difficult to care about anything. Hope is the spark to the blaze of passionate living.

Helping others gives me hope. There's a story about a young man who would walk on the beach each morning. On one morning in particular, he noticed someone in the distance repeatedly bending over to pick something up from the sand, only to toss it into the water. As he drew closer, he could see an older gentleman picking up starfish, tossing them back into the ocean. As the two men approached each other, the young man couldn't help but notice that there were quite a few starfish that had washed ashore. He said to the older man, "There are so many of them. Why even bother? It doesn't really matter." The old man picked up another starfish, looked up at the young man and said, "Well, it matters to this one." Then he tossed it out into the ocean. What may seem insignificant to some is everything to someone else. Remembering this story helps me to never underestimate the hope of even just one.

Overcoming the negativity and the uncaring attitude that the world offers requires persistence and faith.

When we look at the brokenness of our families, our country, or our world, it is easy to see how one can become discouraged and dispirited. Some people even come to question the existence of an all-powerful Creator who would allow such madness. The troubles we face every day can seem too daunting and too painful to even begin to address. Nonetheless, anything with real value causes action, and the first step to starting anything is always the most difficult. In the words of Martin Luther King Jr., "Faith is taking the first step even when you don't see the whole staircase."[7] Overcoming the negativity and the uncaring attitude that the world offers requires persistence and faith. Even Jesus warned his disciples regarding the last days: "Because of the increase of wickedness, the love of most will grow cold, but the one who stands firm to the end will be saved." (Matthew 24:12-13). We can express our faith and love through forgiveness, a word of encouragement, or even just a smile. Find something to be passionate about, even if it is "small" because both words and ideas can change the world.

Food for thought:

Therefore we do not lose heart. Though outwardly we are wasting away, yet inwardly we are being renewed day by day. For our light and momentary troubles are achieving for us an eternal glory that far outweighs them all. So we fix our eyes not on what is seen, but on what is unseen, since what is seen is temporary, but what is unseen is eternal.
2 Corinthians 4:16-18

Let us not become weary in doing good, for at the proper time we will reap a harvest if we do not give up.
Galatians 6:9

Therefore, as we have opportunity, let us do good to all people, especially to those who belong to the family of believers.
Galatians 6:10

Whatever you do, work at it with all your heart, as working for the Lord, not for human masters.
Colossians 3:23

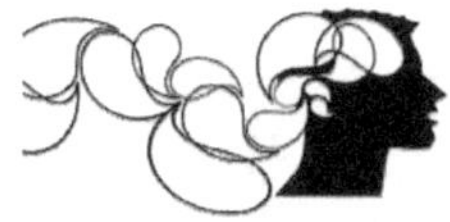

Chapter 3

LET'S TALK ABOUT LOVE

I love you. Three simple words that people long to hear. Love is simple yet profound, daring yet comforting, joyous yet painful, and both desired and dismissed. Most simply put, love is the foundation of the human heart. We all want to express love and be loved in return. We seek it in many places, often not finding it. But love is also a four-letter word. It can break our hearts and make us do things we didn't know we were capable of. Love is contemplated by man more than any other emotion. Thousands of songs have been written in the name of love. We have seen love "lift us up where belong," "keep us together," and even "build a bridge." We have heard that love is "higher," "crazy," "tainted," "bleeding," and, yes, even "groovy." We ask, "How deep is your love?" "Where is the love?" and "What's love got to do with it?" We can think of love as a "crazy little thing" or possibly a "battlefield." Yet even with so many songs written about it, there remains a perplexity about love, questions left unanswered, words left unuttered.

And now these three remain: faith, hope, and love. But the greatest of these is love.

1 Corinthians 13:13

One thing is certain: Love is powerful. When we know that a parent, a spouse or a friend loves us, we feel accepted and valuable. Conversely, a lack of love can make us feel rejected or worthless.

If the imperfect love from fellow human beings is of such great necessity, then the perfect love of our Creator is even more so. God is love and, therefore, an essential presence in our life. Job reminds us that, "Certainly, God is so great that He is beyond our understanding..." (Job 36:26 GWT). Although man may not fathom the complexity of love, we must realize the necessity of it. A Pharisee asked Jesus, "'Teacher, which is the greatest commandment in the Law?' Jesus replied: 'Love the Lord your God with all your heart and with all your soul and with all your mind. This is the first and greatest commandment. And the second is like it. 'Love your neighbor as yourself. All the Law and the Prophets hang on these two commandments'" (Matthew 22:36-40). That means that the love of God, others, and self is the foundation of every principled life. To love God is to get to know Him, and to know Him is to know love. Everything else follows.

JESUS LOVES ME. THIS I KNOW.

God's love is self-sacrificial. Paul tells us, "But for us, there is one God, the Father...and there is one Lord, Jesus Christ, through whom all things were created, and through whom we live" (1 Corinthians 8:6 NLT). All of creation was made through Jesus Christ, and nothing exists apart from him. The Son of God forsook his position in heaven to become flesh, to dwell among us, as one of us. In heaven, He was blessed with the close companionship of his father, enjoyed all that had been made and was especially fond of man. The Bible says that there is no greater love than to lay down one's own life for the sake of another. Because of that love, "We do see Jesus, who was made lower than the angels for a little while, now crowned with glory and honor because He suffered death, so that by the grace of God He might taste death for everyone" (Hebrews 2:9).

Has anyone ever taken a bullet for you, pulled you out of a burning car, or rescued you from drowning? How would you feel about the person who saved you? You probably would be deeply grateful and praise that person for his or her selflessness. You would be amazed that someone cared so deeply for you. Certainly, you would never forget your rescuer. Jesus, prompted by His profound love for you, left his celestial realm to save you. We are told as much in a very familiar passage from the book of John: "For this is how God loved the world: He gave his one and only Son, so that everyone who believes in him will not perish but have eternal life" (John 3:16 NLT). That is the most quoted of all of Scripture, but the depth of sacrifice on the part of God and His only Son are all too often underappreciated.

There is no greater love than to lay one's own life down for the sake of another.

O. Henry provides a perfect example of this kind of self-sacrificing love in the well-known short story, "The Gift of the Magi." Jim and Della were a young married couple, deeply in love, and wished to buy each other the most perfect Christmas gift. Della, who had just $1.87, found a platinum chain for Jim's treasured pocket watch. It was perfect but cost $21. So in order to buy the chain for him, she decided to cut off her long locks of hair and sell them for $20. She was delighted and hoped that Jim would still see her as beautiful, even without her long hair. That night, Della sat at the table with Jim's gift, waiting for him to come home. When Jim saw what Della had done, he was amazed. For he had sold that very pocket watch in order to buy a beautiful set of combs for Della's hair. They now held each other with a newfound realization of just how far the other would go to show their love, and they relished in just how priceless it really was. O. Henry wrote the story in 1905, but it still resonates with people today and has been read in English classrooms across the globe for over 100 years. To love someone enough to sacrifice what means the most to you is, in my opinion, Divine.

No gift we can ever receive in this life can compare to the gift of eternal life that we receive through Jesus Christ. My first car was 1982 Pontiac T-1000, better known as the *Chevette*. As much as I loved that car, it had 125,000 miles on it, the hatchback wouldn't stay open, and the passenger seat was stuck in the upright position. As with most cars, there was always something needing to be fixed. Could you imagine if I were to have been able to take that car and exchange it for a brand new one, not costing me anything but belief that it was possible? Not only that, but the car I was to receive would be in perfect condition, never age, and require absolutely no maintenance. That would truly be unbelievable! That is how eternal life is, a far superior life than this current one. We receive a glorified body that won't be subject to death or pain. We won't experience darkness or loneliness, for God Himself will be our Light and Companion. We will gain greater intimacy with our Creator and Savior. As Revelation promises, "Never again will [we] hunger; never again will [we] thirst. The sun will not beat down on [us], nor any scorching heat. For the Lamb at the center of the throne will be [our] shepherd; He will lead [us] to springs of living water. And God will wipe away every tear from [our] eyes" (Revelation 7:16-17). Through Christ, we are children of God and joint heirs to His kingdom. Only by rejecting Him do we miss out on that provision.

The gift of love in Jesus should evoke in us immense gratitude toward God.

God's love for us is intentional and eternal. It even preceded creation. Paul tells us, "before he made the world, God loved us and chose us in Christ to be holy and without fault in his eyes"(Ephesians 1:4 NLT). David wrote, "What is mankind that you are mindful of them, human beings that you care for them?"(Psalm 8:4). As humans, we typically like to become acquainted with someone or something before claiming our love for it, so the idea that we could be loved prior to our existence is difficult for us to grasp-but no less true. As mothers, we begin to bond with our children long before they are born. Though unheld and unseen, unborn children are genuinely loved by their mothers and that love endures a lifetime. My mother has always been the light of constant love in my life. No matter what I am doing or where I am, she reassures me that I am deeply loved. Her unfailing love for me is priceless. However, God's love is even greater. Isaiah 49:15 reminds us, "Never! Can a mother forget her nursing child? Can she feel no love for the child she has borne? But even if that were possible, I would not forget you!"(NLT)

The door of God's grace is always open.

God Almighty is both the beginning and the end of all things: the one who is, who was, and who is to come (Revelation 1:8). Therefore, there is no moment in our lives when we escape His love. When I look back on some of the dark places I have been in my life, I realize that it was only the love of God that brought me out. In my engagements with the world, I often found myself in situations that potentially could have "taken me out." Yet time and again, God would open his door of grace, via a friend or stranger, and provide "a way out" for me. Like rebellious children, we choose to ignore His loving direction. Like a devoted parent, God never forsakes us. The story of the prodigal son tells us that it was the son who desired to leave his father and that the father allowed him to do so. Upon the son's return, the father rejoiced and embraced him heartily. That is how God loves us. It doesn't matter how far we run or where we try to hide; God is omnipresent. As the Psalmist wrote, "If I go up to the heavens, you are there; if I make my bed in the depths, you are there. If I rise on the wings of the dawn, if I settle on the far side of the sea, even there your hand will guide me, your right hand will hold me fast" (Psalm 139:8-10). He knew me before I was formed in my mother's womb and knows every step I will take but loves me anyway. God's love for me is limitless. The apostle Paul said it this way, "For I am convinced that neither death nor life, neither angels nor principalities, neither the present nor the future, nor any powers, neither height nor depth, nor anything else in all creation, will be able to separate us from the love of God that is in Christ Jesus our Lord." (Romans 8:38-39 BSB). This, I have learned through his faithfulness to me, even during my rebellion.

There is no moment in our lives when we escape His love.

God's love is unchanging and faithful. His Word is true, so we need not fear Him "having second thoughts." For "God is not like people. He tells no lies. He is not like humans. He doesn't change his mind. When he says something, he does it. When he makes a promise, he keeps it" (Numbers 23:19 GWT). No matter where we are, where we have been, or where we are going, the love that our Father has for us is constant and unforced. Poor decisions can lead us to places that are not good for us, but God's love gives us the freedom to choose and He will not take that away. He declares the end from the beginning and promises that the work He has begun in us will be completed. His purpose will be fulfilled. Jesus said, "My Father, who has given them to me, is greater than all, and no one is able to snatch them out of my Father's hand" (John 10:29). His love never fails.

God's love is supernatural and impartial. Science has programmed us to believe Newton's third law of motion, that for every action there is an equal and opposite reaction. Accordingly, some people tend to give love only if it is earned. Even some religions teach that we must somehow merit God's love. That is a lie. Scripture tells us, "But when the kindness and love of God our Savior appeared, He saved us, not because of righteous things we had done, but because of His mercy..."(Titus 3:4-5). His love is a gift, given to the undeserving. It not only transcends time and place but covers all sin. Man can forgive but forgetting is altogether a different story. God's love says that He will remember our sins no more. His love for us does not require us to change in order to receive it. Knowing that we are accepted just as we are is a blessing many seek to find, and God gives us that assurance. Realizing the depth of His love for me has changed me, for the better.

There is an ancient Chinese story about a water bearer who had two clay water pots hanging on either side of his carrying pole. One pot had a crack halfway down its side. Each day, the water bearer would make his journey to the well and fill his pots, and each day, upon his return, he would have one and a half pots of water. This went on for a couple of years. The perfect pot was proud of all it had accomplished, but the cracked pot was ashamed of its imperfection. One day, the cracked pot spoke to the water bearer saying, "I am ashamed of myself because I am cracked. I leak water on the entire trip back home." The water bearer responded with these words, "Did you notice that there were flowers on your side of the path, but not on the other pot's side? I have always known about your flaw, so I planted flower seeds on your side, and every day, while we walk back, you've watered them. For two years, I have been able to pick these beautiful flowers to decorate the table. Without you being just as you are, there would not be beauty to grace the house."

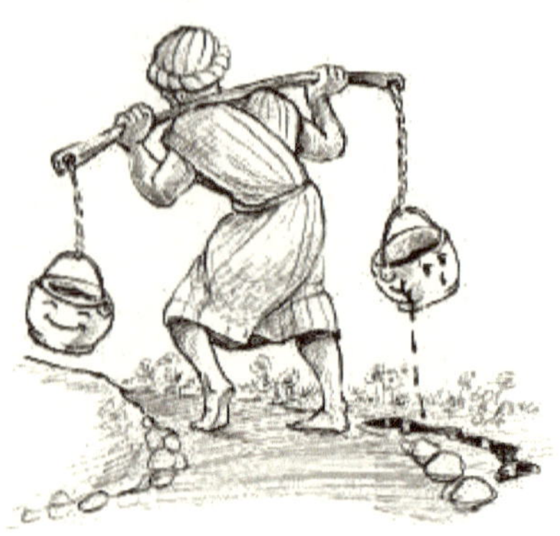

Realizing the depth of His love for me has changed me.

Only God's love for us can reveal our genuine purpose and make all things work together for our good. Trust that it is an extraordinary thing and let it cause you to rejoice. We must remember to "Give thanks to the God of heaven! His loving devotion endures forever" (Psalm 136:26 BSB). It doesn't matter who you are because "He causes His sun to rise upon the evil and the good and sends rain on both the righteous and the unrighteous" (Matthew 5:45 BSB). There is a loving purpose for everyone and everything in creation. He desires all men to be saved and to live eternally with Him. Each of us have equal opportunity to accept this invitation but can only do so by faith. As Paul reminds us, "For by grace you are saved through faith, and this not of yourselves; it is the gift of God" (Ephesians 2:8 BLB).

I'M OKAY. YOU'RE OKAY.

Because God loves us wholeheartedly, we need to learn to love ourselves, too. I believe that most of us have things we don't like about ourselves. I have found that I am my worst critic. I tend to beat myself up over the mistakes I have made, which contradicts the freedom I have found in Christ. Like the cracked pot, we all have flaws, but they are purposeful, and we just don't realize it. That is why listening to God and trusting Him is a vital component of learning to love ourselves.

Some may argue that there is too much self-indulgence in this world, and in certain areas, I would have to agree. It is a dangerous thing to be self-absorbed, thinking only of what benefits you. An "only me" mentality hurts all those around you and is self-destructive. Take, for instance, the Greek mythological character Narcissus, who was deeply loved by a young maiden, who would often follow him through the hills. Narcissus wanted nothing to do with her. It saddened her so deeply that she pined away in grief, until nothing was left of her but her voice. She became simply the echo that could be heard by all who would call out for her in the vast hills. One day, after rejecting Echo, Narcissus was lured to a pool of water, where he saw his own reflection. He fell so deeply in love with it that he refused to tear his gaze away, and he faded into a mere golden flower on the banks of the water. This type of extreme self-love is irrational, but nonetheless, possible. Paul warned us about the last days: "People will be lovers of themselves, lovers of money, boastful, proud, abusive, disobedient to their parents, ungrateful, unholy, without love, unforgiving, slanderous, without self-control, brutal, not lovers of the good, treacherous, rash, conceited, lovers of pleasure rather than lovers of God" (2 Timothy 3:2-4). This type of behavior is harmful.

We must understand that it isn't wrong to love oneself. In fact, healthy love of self is essential. The French Nobel Prize winner, Andre Gide, wrote, "Loving yourself isn't vanity; it is sanity."[1] Certainly, a much more balanced attitude regarding our self is necessary. We live in an aggressive age and, if we aren't standing up for ourselves, we can be easily beaten down. My mother once told me that we must take care of ourselves in order to take care of anyone else and I have found that to be very true. After all, isn't that one of the first instructions airline passengers are given in the event of an emergency? I spent many years neglecting myself, ignoring my need to *matter*. So much so, that I possessed little self-worth and found it difficult to accomplish much good in the world, if any. Lucille Ball said, "Love yourself first and everything else falls in line. You really have to love yourself to get anything done in this world."[2] To love ourselves sensibly, it is important to view ourselves through God's lens and not our own. As Paul told the Corinthians, it would be beneficial for us to "Examine [ourselves], to see whether [we] are in the faith" (2 Corinthians 13:5). Such examination and self-reflection are keys to a healthy sense of self-esteem.

Healthy love of self is essential.

Receiving God's unconditional love makes us a vessel for his love. In Romans, Paul writes, "through whom also we have access by faith into this grace in which we stand...because the love of God has been poured out into our hearts through the

Holy Spirit, the One having been given to us (Romans 5:2,5 BLB). We are compelled to reflect that love towards others by the power of the Holy Spirit, and it is only by that same power that we can do so without reservation. Jesus, Himself, set the definition of love by personifying it for us. He became Love in the flesh. In the well-known "love" chapter of 1 Corinthians, Paul gives us a sort of "checklist" concerning love: "Love is patient, love is kind. It does not envy, it does not boast, it is not proud. It does not dishonor others, it is not self-seeking, it is not easily angered, it keeps no record of wrongs. Love does not delight in evil but rejoices with the truth. It always protects, always trusts, always hopes, always perseveres" (13:4-7). We are commanded to love one another just as God has loved us (John 15:12). Being patient, kind, humble and forgiving may sound practical enough when we are dealing with a child, spouse, parent or friend. But, what about complete strangers or even our enemies? Jesus said, "If you love only those who love you, what reward is there for that? Even corrupt tax collectors do that much. If you are kind only to your friends, how are you different from anyone else? Even pagans do that. But you are to be perfect, even as your Father in heaven is perfect" (Matthew 5:46-48 NLT). The Greek word here for *perfect* actually means "to be complete." We are not being commanded to never make mistakes, but to reach a level of greater maturity by loving others without partiality.

Foregoing self-interests and forgiving others are essential habits to possess if we are to walk in love.

During his sermon on the mount, Jesus said, "But I say, love your enemies. Pray for those who persecute you" (Matthew 5:44 NLT). It is not as easy as it sounds. When we are treated unfairly, our initial response is to retaliate, taking vengeance into our own hands. However, that only leads to more adversity. I spent years in civil court, in opposition to my children's father, pointing fingers and defending myself, playing the character assassination game. All to no avail. The judge eventually decided that trying to mediate was impossible and ruled against joint *anything,* based on the parties' inability to communicate. As a result, distance between my children and I, inevitably grew. Dismissing the offender and ignoring the problem doesn't help either, it only seeks to disguise it temporarily. It will eventually rear its ugly head at another time. The best way to resolve the matter is to invite God into the situation. We do so by taking a more proactive approach. Conquer the evil with the good. Jesus instructed: "If you are sued in court and your shirt is taken from you, give your coat, too. If a soldier demands that you carry his gear for a mile, carry it two miles. Give to those who ask, and don't turn away from those who want to borrow" (Matthew 5:40-42 NLT). A couple of years ago my husband and I started to send a Christmas card with a gift card inside to my children's father. It may sound like a simple thing, but doing so was not that easy. We stepped out in faith, and though we have no way of knowing how that simple act may affect his life, we know that God has blessed us in our obedience and that he is in God's hands. There is great peace in that. By loving our enemies, we show them the surpassing power of good over evil. Paul further explains this idea in his letter to Rome: "If your enemy is hungry, feed him; if he is thirsty, give him something to drink. In doing this, you will heap burning coals on his head" (Romans 12:20). Those "burning coals" will demand his attention and hopefully direct him towards God, who is Love.

Foregoing self-interests and forgiving others are essential habits to possess if we are to walk in love. Jesus illustrates what loving our neighbors is like in the story of the good Samaritan. When Jesus spoke of the man who had been robbed, he said that he "fell among robbers, and they stripped him and beat him, and went away leaving him half dead" (Luke 10:30 NASB). By describing the man as unable to speak and naked, the two identifying factors were eliminated. Therefore, there was no way for anyone passing by to know the man's ethnicity or status. The first two passersby did not attempt to find out whether or not the man was a fellow Jew or even alive. They were too self-concerned and preoccupied. Similarly, our busyness can prevent us from taking advantage of opportunities to show love to others. Conversely, the Samaritan showed true love, which requires attention, compassion, time, and sometimes, even resources. Like the Samaritan, we should seek to look beyond superficial circumstance and not allow our own bias to prevent us from acknowledging human need.

No one is more significant than another.

A young college senior had just sat down to take his final exam. The last question was, "What is the janitor's name?" He was quick to raise his hand and ask the professor if it were a real question that would be scored. The professor readily said, "Yes." He then added, "In this life, whatever you do, you will be around people. No one is more significant than another. It is important to acknowledge them all equally and to never underestimate their worth." That student learned a valuable life lesson even though he didn't know the janitor's name—Dorothy.

Love is much more than just an emotion, an act of kindness, or a giving of yourself. It is a condition of the heart, which affects how we behave in every aspect of our lives. We love because He first loved us and are called to be His children: "See how great a love the Father has bestowed on us, that we would be called children of God; and such we are" (1 John 3:1

NASB). God operates by love and, because we are created in his image, we are beckoned to do the same. Thankfully God has graced us with power from on high that accomplishes more than what is within our human ability (Acts 1:8). Realizing that we all share this big wide world enables us to be more open to loving one another. Understanding that God has given us all that we have helps us to be more generous. Choosing to love even when it is difficult keeps us close to God. We are able to "come to know and to believe the love that God has for us..." and that "whoever abides in love abides in God, and God in him" (1 John 4:16 BSB). Love is above all things and outside of love exists no substantial thing. Paul reminds us of the supremacy of love in 1 Corinthians 13:1-3:

> *If I speak in the tongues of men or of angels, but do not have love, I am only a resounding gong or a clanging cymbal. If I have the gift of prophecy and can fathom all mysteries and all knowledge, and if I have a faith that can move mountains, but do not have love, I am nothing. If I give all I possess to the poor and give over my body to hardship that I may boast, but do not have love, I gain nothing.*

So, let us strive to live...and let love prevail!

Chapter 4

CAN'T TOUCH THIS—
THE GRANDEUR OF GOD

You are in a crowded restaurant. Notice all the people, the lights, the sounds, the smell. Absorb the moment. Think about the fact that all of this is happening on a massive rock-like ball suspended in mid-air. Furthermore, this ball is spinning at an equatorial speed of 1,000 mph while it orbits the sun at 66,640 mph! Does anyone seem to be affected by this? No. Life just goes on while the miraculous power of our existence is at work, 24 hours a day, 365 days a year.

God's very name, Jehovah, differentiates Him as the self-existing God. He is the Alpha and the Omega, the beginning of all of creation. Nothing exists apart from Him, and He is eternal. He is the Great I Am and alone sits high above the earth (Isaiah 40:22). As such, nothing compares to Him. In the book of Genesis, we read that God merely spoke and things came into existence (Genesis 1). His very words are powerful; they evoke action: "So is my word that goes out from my mouth: It will not return to me empty, but will accomplish what I desire and achieve the purpose for which I sent it" (Isaiah 55:11). He intentionally designs all things prior to their creation, and His plan is perfect and sovereign.

Romans 1:20 tells us, "From the creation of the world, God's invisible qualities, his eternal power and divine nature, have been clearly observed in what he made."(GWT) It only takes a minute to witness nature and see the handiwork of our creative designer. From the tiniest microorganism to the grandest galaxy, creation declares the majesty of its maker. Taking time to "smell the flowers" is taking time to get to know God. His perfect construction has been mimicked by man in science, medicine, and engineering. Everywhere we look, we can see echoes of His hand. Common Velcro was invented by copying the characteristics of the annoying burr. Swimsuits and boats are now being made with "sharkskin" technology in order to increase speed and efficiency. Even "smart" cities and data-based systems are designed based on the organizational skills of the humble bee. Some of the world's greatest inventors attribute the design of their inventions to the creativity of God. George Washington Carver, the famous Peanut Man, said, "I love to think of nature as an unlimited broadcasting station, through which God speaks to us every hour, if we will only tune in."[1]

> *The important thing is to take the time to listen to God's voice, His word, and His creation.*

We are also a part of God's creation and built with amazing detail. For instance, the human nose can detect over 50,000 scents and the human eye can distinguish over 10 million different colors! If we were to uncoil the DNA within our body, it would reach to Pluto and back. The human body has been studied for centuries and yet there is always something new to discover about it. God has also seen fit to impart some of that great ingenuity into our minds and hearts so that we, too, can take part in the joy of creating. The inventor of the laser printer, Gary Starkweather said, "I believe that to a great extent, the creativity we possess is because the Creator put it there."[2]

THAT'S SO AWESOME

God's watermark is also found in His written word. The Book of Job highlights God's matchless power and infinite wisdom. The first thirty-seven chapters relay many of man's assumptions and their attempts to explain God. When God finally responds in chapter 38, His distinct supremacy is revealed:

> Then the Lord spoke to Job out of the storm.
> He said:
> "Where were you when I laid the earth's foundation?
> Tell me, if you understand.
> Who marked off its dimensions?
> Surely you know!
> Who stretched a measuring line across it?
> On what were its footings set,
> or who laid its cornerstone—
> while the morning stars sang together
> and all the angels shouted for joy?
> "Who shut up the sea behind doors
> when it burst forth from the womb,
> when I made the clouds its garment
> and wrapped it in thick darkness,
> when I fixed limits for it
> and set its doors and bars in place,
> when I said, 'This far you may come and no farther;
> here is where your proud waves halt'?
> "Have you ever given orders to the morning,
> or shown the dawn its place?
> (Job 38:4-12)

God continues to ask Job over fifty different questions regarding His creation—all of which are worth pondering ourselves. Do you know where light and darkness live? Have you walked the depths of the sea or seen the gates of death? Can you cause stars to appear in the sky or seasons to change? Can you lead the bear and its cubs out of their den in due time? How is it that the rooster understands the day? Why is the ostrich mighty yet not so wise? Why does the horse stomp the ground before charging and run at the blast of a trumpet? God goes into great detail proving to Job that He alone is aware of all living things and sustains all life. Job is silenced yet continues to listen:

God said:

"Look at Behemoth,

which I made along with you

and which feeds on grass like an ox.

What strength it has in its loins,

what power in the muscles of its belly!

Its tail sways like a cedar;

the sinews of its thighs are close-knit.

Its bones are tubes of bronze,

its limbs like rods of iron.

It ranks first among the works of God,

yet its Maker can approach it with his sword.

The hills bring it their produce,

and all the wild animals play nearby.

Under the lotus plants it lies,

hidden among the reeds in the marsh.

The lotuses conceal it in their shadow;

the poplars by the stream surround it.

A raging river does not alarm it;

it is secure, though the Jordan should surge against its mouth.

Can anyone capture it by the eyes or trap it and pierce its nose?

(Job 40:15-24)

"Can you pull in Leviathan with a fishhook
or tie down its tongue with a rope?
Can you put a cord through its nose
or pierce its jaw with a hook?
Will it keep begging you for mercy?
Will it speak to you with gentle words?
Will it make an agreement with you
for you to take it as your slave for life?
Can you make a pet of it like a bird
or put it on a leash for the young women
 in your house?
Will traders barter for it?
Will they divide it up among the merchants?
Can you fill its hide with harpoons
or its head with fishing spears?
If you lay a hand on it,
you will remember the struggle and never
do it again!
Any hope of subduing it is false;
the mere sight of it is overpowering.
No one is fierce enough to rouse it.
Who then is able to stand against me?
Who has a claim against me that I must pay?
Everything under heaven belongs to me.
(Job 41:1-11)

Job was astounded by God's vast wisdom, and he realized that there was so much in this world that he could just not fathom. He was left in complete awe and, in being so, came to humbly accept his place in creation. There's no better way for us to be awe-inspired than to spend time watching a sunset or a starry sky, to witness God's creatures in all their diversity, or to see the seasons revealing their splendor. Then maybe we can come to echo Job's words to God:

"I know that you can do all things;
no purpose of yours can be thwarted...
Surely, I spoke of things I did not understand,
things too wonderful for me to know...
My ears had heard of you
but now my eyes have seen you."
(Job 42:2-3,5)

THE MADMAN

In the story of Jonah, we learn that God's plans are absolute. After Jonah's dramatic rescue from the big fish, he obediently went to preach destruction upon the city of Nineveh. When the people heard Jonah, they all repented, and God did not destroy them. Jonah felt foolish. He didn't want the people saved. He saw God's decision as wrong and was frustrated and angry with God. So, he built himself a shelter just outside of the city and sat down to watch what would happen to Nineveh.

He pleaded with God, saying "...it is better
for me to die than to live."(Jonah 4:3)

But God said to him, "Is it right for you to be
angry?" (Jonah 4:4)

God made a leafy plant to grow so that it gave Jonah shade and made him more comfortable. For that, Jonah was glad. However, the next day God sent a worm to chew on the plant and it wilted. When the sun came out, it burned Jonah's head. Jonah again complained about his plight: "It would be better for me to die than to live."(Jonah 4:8) His comment set off an important conversation:

> *Then God said to Jonah, "Is it right for you to be angry because the plant died?"*

> *"Yes," Jonah retorted, " even angry enough to die!"*

> *Then the LORD said, "You feel sorry about the plant, though you did nothing to put it there. It came quickly and died quickly. But Nineveh has more than 120,000 people living in spiritual darkness, not to mention all the animals. Shouldn't I feel sorry for such a great city?"*

> *(Jonah 4:9-11 NLT)*

I can relate to Jonah. I've found myself questioning God many times, especially when things aren't going the way I think they should. It is in those times when I remind myself that my perspective is limited and that my emotions may be clouding my ability to trust God's "big picture." Isaiah tells us that God's thoughts are not our thoughts and that His ways are not ours. In God's own words, "As the heavens are higher than the earth, so are my ways higher than your ways and my thoughts than your thoughts" (Isaiah 55:9). As He did with Jonah, God must sometimes remind us that He is in charge and that we, despite our opinion to the contrary, are not.

I'VE SEEN FIRE AND I'VE SEEN RAIN

Ezra complained to God about mankind. He blamed God for the existence of evil men, saying, "Yet thou didst not take away from them their evil heart..."(2 Esdras 3:20 KJV). Ezra is so distraught that he condemns God for sparing the wicked and for not showing man how to comprehend His ways. He even accuses God of forsaking His people and finding another. Ezra asks, "Or has another nation known thee besides Israel?"(2 Esdras 3:32 KJV). When Ezra finishes his prayer, God sends an angel to reply to him:

> *Then the angel said to me, "Your understanding has utterly failed regarding this world, and do you think you can comprehend the way of the Most High?" Then I said, "Yes, my lord." And he replied to me, "I have been sent to show you three ways, and to put before you three problems. If you can solve one of them for me, I also will show you the way you desire to see and will teach you why the heart is evil." I said, "Speak on, my lord." And he said to me, "Go, weigh for me the weight of fire, or measure for me a measure of wind, or call back for me the day that is past." I answered and said, "Who of those that have been born can do this, that you ask me concerning these things?" And he said to me, "If I had asked you, 'How many dwellings are in the heart of the sea, or how many streams are at the source of the deep, or how many streams are above the firmament, or which are the exits of hell, or which are the entrances of paradise?' Perhaps you would have said to me, 'I never went down into the deep, nor as yet into hell, neither did I ever ascend into heaven.' But now I have asked you only*

about fire and wind and the day, things through which you have passed and without which you cannot exist, and you have given me no answer about them!" And he said to me, "You cannot understand the things with which you have grown up; how then can your mind comprehend the way of the Most High? And how can one who is already worn out by the corrupt world understand incorruption?" When I heard this, I fell on my face and said to him, "It would be better for us not to be here than to come here and live in ungodliness, and to suffer and not understand why." (2 Esdras 4:1-11 RSV)

The angel's message is certainly poignant, and Ezra's position relatable. There are many things that we live with day in and day out, yet we cannot understand them. For example, years of effort have gone into attempting to eradicate poverty, disease, and famine. Yet, we still haven't eliminated them. If we cannot figure that out, how can we possibly figure God out? We shouldn't fault ourselves for not being able to do so. It's just the way that it is. God knows man's limitations for He said, "Even the stork in the sky knows her seasons; and the turtledove and the swift and the thrush observe the time of their migration; but My people do not know the ordinance of the Lord" (Jeremiah 8:7 NASB).

The important thing is to take the time to listen to God's voice, His word, and His creation. Remembering the story of Mary and Martha helps me do just that. Jesus had come to visit, and Martha stayed busy trying to prepare, but Mary sat down at Jesus' feet to hear Him speak. Martha, feeling the burden of the work, grew upset and asked Jesus to tell Mary to help her. "But the Lord answered and said to her, 'Martha, Martha, you are worried and bothered about so many things; but *only* one thing is necessary, for Mary has chosen the good part, which shall not be taken away from her.'" (Luke 10:41-42 NASB). In other words, paying attention to God is of utmost importance. Coming to know God as *the grand maestro of the universe* better equips us to not only sit at His feet and listen but to join the ensemble. We can say, as the Psalmist did:

> *"Many, O LORD my God, are the wonders which You have done, And Your thoughts toward us; There is none to compare with You. If I would declare and speak of them, they would be too numerous to count."*

> *(Psalm 40:5 NASB)*

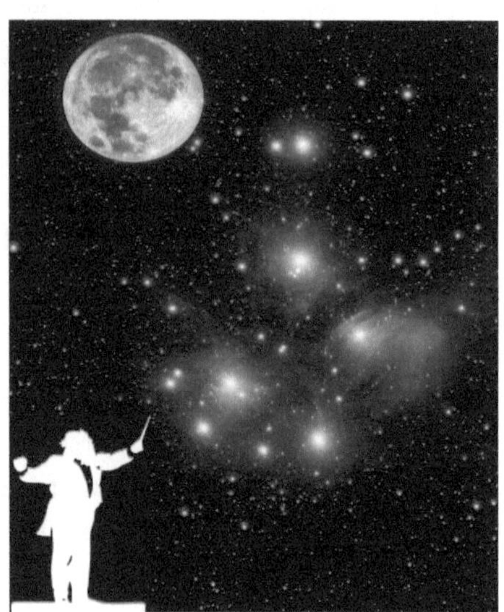

©Your Light Publishing

Chapter 5

THERE'S SOMETHING ABOUT JESUS

One Solitary Life

He was born in an obscure village, the child of a peasant. He grew up in another village, where he worked in a carpenter shop until he was 30. Then, for three years, he was an itinerant preacher.

He never wrote a book. He never held an office. He never had a family or owned a home. He didn't go to college. He never lived in a big city. He never traveled 200 miles from the place where he was born. He did none of the things that usually accompany greatness. He had no credentials but himself.

He was only 33 when the tide of public opinion turned against him. His friends ran away. One of them denied him. He was turned over to his enemies and went through the mockery of a trial. He was nailed to a cross between two thieves. While he was dying, his executioners gambled for his garments, the only property he had on earth. When he was dead, he was laid in a borrowed grave, through the pity of a friend.

Twenty centuries have come and gone, and today he is the central figure of the human race. I am well within the mark when I say that all the armies that ever marched, all the navies that ever sailed, all the parliaments that ever sat, all the kings that ever reigned--put together--have not affected the life of man on this earth as much as that one, solitary life.

Attributed to James Allen Francis.

I remember reading those words for the first time. After my father died, I would often walk the grounds of the cemetery where he was buried, in search of inner peace. I came across a large stone plaque engraved with the words of that poem. Simply reading them engraved them upon my heart as well. What impacted me the most was that there was no mention of a name within its lines, but there was little doubt about whom the author was speaking. It was at that moment that I realized how much I needed Jesus to be the paramount figure of my spiritual life. As a result of that decision, I have come to see Jesus in both simple and profound ways, but most importantly as the perfect reflection of God.

My father was a navy chief for many years. As such, structure and character were important to him, and he wanted to instill them in his own children. House rules were posted with "taps" at a certain time and time limits set on the use of the phone and TV. There were consequences —sometimes unorthodox— for disobedience. Once my sister and I were made to wash the dishes while blindfolded because we were evidently making fun of being blind. His aim was to implement discipline for our own good, but it was often misunderstood. My dad would occasionally take me to work with him on the naval base. He showed me how lasers worked and gave me tours of the airplane hangars. Witnessing his work and seeing his comrades saluting him taught me that there is a great reward in hard work. He even took me on a short cruise on the aircraft carrier, U.S.S. America. On that cruise I somehow wandered off and found myself below deck, staring frighteningly out at the big blue ocean waves. A young sailor saw my fear and led me back to my dad. Taking hold of my father's hand calmed my fear and put my heart at ease. As I grew older, I didn't want that same closeness. While praying "The Our Father" at church, the congregation would hold hands. When the prayer was over, my dad would continue to hold my hand as if to remind me that I was never alone and that I was loved. I didn't appreciate that then; I only wish I had. As a parent myself, I too want to hold my children's hands forever. I want them to feel loved and to have more opportunities than I ever had. I wish I could infuse them with everything I've learned in life so that they wouldn't have to struggle so much in order to figure it all out. My dad was more of a doer than a talker. He was more apt to spend time with you building something in his workshop than to sit down and discuss something. This trait impressed upon me the reality that actions speak louder than words. There are many things I "picked up" from my father that I didn't realize until I was much older. I only wish I would have taken more advantage of the time I had with my dad. Maybe I would have learned a little more. At the same time, I am grateful to have received such fatherly provision, guidance, discipline, and love from my dad for as long as I did.

OUR FATHER WHO ART IN HEAVEN

Although our earthly fathers hold a special and important role in our lives, it is still only temporary. As our *Everlasting Father,*

Jesus' provision, guidance, discipline, and love is complete and endures forever. He accomplishes this by presenting Himself with many different "faces" and in different ways.

The Lord is My Shepherd

A shepherd is responsible for tending his sheep, feeding them, leading them to water and letting them graze in green pastures. As "sheep," we are cared for by our "shepherd" in much the same way. Of course, reading the Bible is one way for us to be fed and refreshed, but sometimes we are provided for more miraculously. Some years ago, I was a few hundred dollars short for my next month's rent. I had just left a church service and was approaching my car when I saw that there was an envelope taped to the window. I opened it to find a few hundred dollars in cash inside. I don't know who on earth put that money there for me, but I know that it was because of the loving attention of Jesus.

A *good shepherd* searches out his lost sheep. There was a period of my life when I was mad at God, didn't want to read the Bible, and was living in rebellion, I was lost. It was then that He sent the man who would become my husband into my life. When we met, he made me laugh and wanted genuine companionship. He spoke of how he loved God and wanted to understand the Bible. It was through that relationship that Jesus sought me and found me.

Shepherds also protect their flock. It is common even today to come across small openings in the caves throughout the mountains in the middle east. At night or during bad weather, the shepherd would lead his flock into the shelter and then lay across the opening as a "gate." This made sure that the sheep would not go out and that nothing could come in without the shepherd's knowing. Jesus told his followers, "Truly, truly, I tell you, I am the gate for the sheep" (John 10:7 BSB). His faithful presence as our guard brings us comfort and security. Just like my wandering away from my dad on the ship placed me in a frightening place, wandering away from our heavenly father's direction puts us in a fearful, unprotected place. Being obedient to his voice and abiding in his love keeps us safe.

Keep Calm and Seek Him

For centuries, people have used the starry skies to guide them. The brightest star, Sirius, is used as the point of reference upon which to navigate a journey. That same star shines brightly enough to remain visible in the sky right up until daylight. Seeing that star also means that a new day is on the horizon. Consequently, it is called the Morning Star. It is not coincidence that Revelation calls Jesus *"the Bright and Morning Star."* Jesus is the "star" by which we are to navigate our lives. I have traveled in the dark, both physically and spiritually. Both are dangerous places to be, especially if you have lost your way. Seeing the light of Jesus' love in every circumstance helps to direct me to the right path and gives me the confidence that a new day is coming. Paul reminds us, "Therefore if anyone is in Christ, he is a new creation. The old has passed away. Behold, the new has come!" (2 Corinthians 5:17 BSB). Now that I've been found, I keep my eyes fixed on Jesus as I journey through this life.

The light of Jesus is no ordinary light. It reaches into the hearts and minds of men. As *Rabbi*, He taught from boats, in the synagogues, and on the streets. When He spoke, he captured peoples' attention with the words He spoke. Matthew reports that "When Jesus had finished saying these things, the crowds were amazed at his teaching, for he taught with real authority— quite unlike their teachers of religious law" (Matthew 7:28-29 NLT). It was the bright light from heaven, Jesus, who blinded Saul on the road to Damascus. That light surrounded him, made him fall to the ground, and immediately converted him (Acts 22:6-11). I have listened to many teachers, motivational speakers, pastors, world leaders, and self-help gurus. Although I find their words helpful to a degree, I always end up with more questions. None of them teach me as completely or as powerfully as Jesus. His ability to interject parables and use simple short stories to teach profound lessons makes them both understandable and memorable.

The light of Jesus is no ordinary light.

My twenties and thirties were rather turbulent times for me. Raising kids, developing relationships, tracking finances, and working each day was all very difficult for me to manage. Reflecting on simple memories of my dad just didn't seem to suffice; I longed for his personal advice. That, of course, wasn't possible. Many of us are in this situation because our earthly fathers are absent from us. However, we do have a direct line to our *Heavenly Father* through prayer. Isaiah 9:6 reminds us that we have a *Counselor* in Him: "For to us a child is born, to us a son is given, and the government will be on his shoulders. And he will be called Wonderful Counselor, Mighty God, Everlasting Father, Prince of Peace." Jesus is wise, able to read even the hearts of all men. Today, men of power strive to gain advisers with such beneficial insight. Yet no man's advice can compare to the wisdom of Jesus. I consider it a privilege to have Him as my Counselor. He never fails to bring understanding to my confusion.

The more I learn from Him, the more I want to learn. Paul directs us to "have the full riches of complete understanding, in order that we may know the mystery of God, namely, Christ, in whom are hidden all the treasures of wisdom and knowledge" (Colossians 2:8 BSB). The more we seek these "treasures," the more we learn about ourselves and our relationship to God.

Learn to Love Copycatting

Most people find that being copied is annoying. But mimicry is really just a reflection of admiration. Children love to mimic the behavior of others, especially their parents. I did this often. I used to love dressing up like them and pretending to do what they did. When I was much younger, I enjoyed games which required me to copy what I saw or heard, such as "Simon Says" and "Follow the Leader." It was a part of my everyday life. I didn't realize then that imitation is a powerful tool of influence. There's no greater way to teach a child than to set an example for them to follow.

Jesus came to earth to be our *example*. His words, "Follow me," are actually a command. However, the Greek word for following is not "passive." It's more than just a simple game of following the leader. It indicates that the follower is assisting or actively participating in the task at hand. It requires us to learn from Jesus' actions and duplicate them by taking part in the work He did. His work revolved around people. He went through all the towns and villages, teaching in the synagogues, proclaiming the good news of the Kingdom and healing every disease and sickness. His compassion for these people drove His life. He saw the people as harassed and helpless, like sheep without a shepherd. He said to his disciples, "The harvest is plentiful, but the workers are few. Ask the Lord of the harvest, therefore, to send out workers into his harvest field" (Matthew 9:35-38). We can share in the work of harvesting souls. First, by feeling compassion for others and then by expressing it. Peter said, "For God called you to do good, even if it means suffering, just as Christ suffered for you. He is your example, and you must follow in his steps" (1 Peter 2:21 NLT).

A picture is worth a thousand words and one of the most powerful images I have seen is the one of Jesus washing the feet of his disciples. Jesus, who called us to be servants, first showed us how to be one. He said this: "You call me 'Teacher' and 'Lord,' and rightly so, for that is what I am. Now that I, your Lord and Teacher, have washed your feet, you also should wash one another's feet. I have set you an example that you should do as I have done for you" (John 13:13-15). Imitating Christ assures us that we remain in Him and in love, for "the one who says he abides in Him ought himself to walk in the same manner as He walked" (1 John 2:6 NASB). By His example, we are taught what it truly means to "love one another."

Suffer the pain of discipline or suffer the pain of regret.

Knowing right from wrong takes time and—often—requires making mistakes. As a teenager, I used to hang out with my friends and just drive around. Some of my friends had pick-up trucks, and my father had told me to never ride in the back. However, one day my friends and I were coming back from the beach, and I decided to hop in the back for the ride home. We had an accident, and I literally flipped out and slid across the asphalt on my bottom. I received first, second, and third degree burns from my heels to my hips. Needless to say, I realized my stupidity in disobeying my dad and was dreading what lay ahead, but the humiliation, the pain, and the long-term recovery, in itself, were discipline enough. My parents just loved me through it. Jesus treats us much the same way.

***His judgment is fair and trustworthy,
and He alone holds the right to judge.***

We all appear before the judgment seat of Christ because he is *Judge* of both the living and the dead: "For not even the Father judges anyone, but He has given all judgment to the Son" (John 5:22 NASB). Isaiah tells us, "He will not judge by what he sees with his eyes or decide by what he hears with his ears; but with righteousness he will judge the needy, with justice he will give decisions for the poor of the earth" (Isaiah 11:3-4). Love prompted Jesus to come to earth to bring us the opportunity for eternal life. But along with that, He brought judgment. John gives us this reminder: "And this is the verdict: The Light has come into the world, but men loved the darkness rather than the Light because their deeds were evil" (John 3:19 BSB). His judgment is fair and trustworthy, and He alone holds the right to judge. We are admonished, "Do not complain, brethren, against one another, so that you yourselves may not be judged; behold, the Judge is standing right at the door" (James 5:9 NASB).

I'LL BE THERE FOR YOU

My husband is my best friend. We talk, hold hands, work together, and are very rarely apart. He takes care of me and makes me feel special. When we are not with each other, I feel like something is missing. Some people long for that type of relationship, spending an awful lot of time being alone. Though Jesus may not physically hold our hands, He does love us in the same way a groom cares for his bride. Speaking in response to the Pharisees, who were condemning His disciples for not fasting, He said, "How can the guests of the bridegroom mourn while he is with them? The time will come when the bridegroom will be taken from them; then they will fast"(Matthew 9:15). He cherishes and honors his bride, who is the church. He lays his own life down for the sake of having his bride upon His return. That is a real friend and true love. We can have an intimate relationship with Jesus in this life as we wait for the day to arrive when we will certainly "rejoice and be glad and give Him glory! For the wedding of the Lamb has come, and His bride has made herself ready" (Revelation 19:7).

Jesus is also a friend who gives us lasting comfort. Joseph Scriven, an Irish poet, was engaged to a young lady whom he had loved for quite some time. But shortly before the wedding day arrived, his promised bride died, and he fell into deep sorrow. Through his sad experience, he realized his own dependency upon Christ and was compelled to write the poem, "What a Friend We Have in Jesus." It is now a well-known hymn:

What a friend we have in Jesus,
all our sins and griefs to bear! What a
privilege to carry
everything to God in prayer!
O what peace we often forfeit,
O what needless pain we bear,
all because we do not carry
everything to God in prayer.
Have we trials and temptations?
Is there trouble anywhere?
We should never be discouraged;
take it to the Lord in prayer.
Can we find a friend so faithful
who will all our sorrows share?
Jesus knows our every weakness;
take it to the Lord in prayer.
Are we weak and heavy laden,
cumbered with a load of care?
Precious Savior, still our refuge;
take it to the Lord in prayer.
Do thy friends despise, forsake thee?
Take it to the Lord in prayer!
In his arms he'll take and shield thee;
thou wilt find a solace there.[1]

Jesus said that He no longer calls us servants, but friends. Proverbs tells us that "a friend loves at all times" (Proverbs 17:17) and that there is a "friend who sticks closer than a brother" (Proverbs 18:24). Jesus is that perfect friend to me. He is with me through thick and thin and will be with me forever. In Matthew, we see His promise to us: "And remember that I am always with you until the end of time"(Matthew 28:20 GWT).

Peaceful Easy Feeling

Even the raging seas obey Jesus' command to "Peace, be still" (Mark 4:39 KJV). So, too, will the storms of our life be calmed when we submit them to Jesus. His promise to us is clear: "Peace I leave with you; my peace I give you. I do not give to you as the world gives. Do not let your hearts be troubled and do not be afraid" (John 14:27). Life inevitably brings situations of disruption. However, the mere presence of the *Prince of Peace* quiets them all. I have seen this fulfilled in my own life, time and time again.

When my infant son was recovering from surgery in the intensive care unit, he had difficulty breathing. A respiratory therapist was working with him when, suddenly, alarms starting ringing, lights began to flash, and nurses stormed the room. I knew that something was devastatingly wrong. I felt shocked and helpless. I looked over at my father-in-law, who happened to be sitting in a chair in the corner of the room. The look on his face was one of complete calm, as if he had the utmost confidence that everything was going to be just fine. His presence at that very moment helped me maintain composure, even after we were escorted out of the room. In his presence, I felt peace. Similarly, we gain an inner peace that surpasses understanding when we dwell in Jesus Christ.

Calming the chaos that erupts in this life is one thing. But what about the relentless hostility that presents itself on the world stage? Remember "For God so loved the world that He gave His one and only son..."(John 3:16) in order " to reconcile to Himself all things, whether things on earth or things in heaven, by making peace through the blood of His cross" (Colossians 1:20 BSB). The Son of God was sent to offer eternal life to those who exercise faith in it. "For he himself is our peace, who has made the two groups one and has destroyed the barrier, the dividing wall of hostility" (Ephesians 2:14). He has bridged the gap between God and men, Jew and Gentile, sinner and saint. I have often wondered, if He has the power to calm every storm, why He doesn't. The bottom line for me is that there is a great divide among men, believers and unbelievers. It is an individual choice to welcome and enter into that "peace agreement" or reject it.

We gain an inner peace that surpasses understanding when we dwell in Jesus Christ.

When you sign any written agreement, you are agreeing with the terms laid out within it. The aforementioned "agreement" between God and man is not on paper. It is made valid by your faith, not your signature. Jesus said, "I am *the way* and *the truth* and *the life*. No one comes to the Father except through me" (John 14:6). Believing that only Jesus leads to communion with God is the way to gain eternal life. He is the truth because He is the perfect image of God. John said, "We have seen his glory, glory as of the only Son from the Father, full of grace and truth" (John 1:14 BSB). Jesus gives eternal life, and he sustains this life, as well. He satisfies our every need. When we believe in Him, we will "never go hungry…and…never be thirsty" (John 6:35). This, He has promised.

HOLDING OUT FOR A HERO

During the time of Jesus, the High Priest was the highest spiritual leader of the Jews. There were many priests, but only one High Priest. His sacred assignment was exclusive to him and highly revered. Once a year, on the day of Atonement, the High Priest would enter the holiest of holies on behalf of all the people. That place was beyond the veil that hung between the Holy and the Most Holy Place. The Most Holy Place was not only the location of the Ark of the Covenant but was where the people believed the presence of God to be. So, entering the holiest of holies meant that the High Priest was actually meeting with God. He would sprinkle the blood offering from the sacrifice upon the mercy seat of the ark, as an effort to make amends for the sin of all the people. When his task was completed all of Israel rejoiced, for now they had a "clean slate" and a right standing with God.

In those days, there were two things needed to accomplish this cleansing: an unblemished sacrificial animal—typically a goat or a lamb, —and one to offer the sacrifice to God. Jesus became both in a more superior way. The blood of animals had to be offered over and over. Jesus was the perfect *Lamb of God* brought to the altar of sacrifice on behalf of all mankind. He presented himself, upon the cross, as a final and everlasting offering to God, saying, "Father, into your hands I commit my spirit" (Luke 23:46). With those words, He eliminated the need for any other sacrifice. It is now through Jesus that we gain access to God. That is why the curtain of the temple was torn in two when Jesus uttered, "It is finished" (John 19:30). Only by Jesus' shed blood are we found acceptable in the sight of God, "For there is one God, and one mediator also between God and men, the man Christ Jesus"(1 Timothy 2:5 NASB). Because we have a "great *High Priest* who has entered heaven, Jesus the Son of God," we are to "hold firmly to what we believe" (Heb. 4:14 NLT). The supreme sacrifice of the blood of the Lamb has made us worthy to do so.

As John Newton, the writer of "Amazing Grace," was dying at age eighty-two, he whispered to a friend, "My memory is nearly gone. But I remember two things: that I am a great sinner, and that Christ is a great Saviour."[2] How simple and true. During the Christmas season, we typically hear this verse, "For unto you is born this day in the city of David a Saviour, who is Christ the Lord" (Luke 2:11 KJV). The thought of this baby boy in a manger conjures up deep sentiment, but what does it mean to be a Saviour?

Through Christ, we are free from the stain of sin and the sting of death.

The question "are you saved?" is often used in Christianity, but it is also under-defined. The idea of being "saved" can be an unclear notion. You can "save" money or a piece of cake by setting it aside for safe-keeping. You "save" a trip by preventing a needless one. A "save" can even be the play that keeps the opponent from scoring. More importantly, a medic can "save" a life by performing CPR. Jesus Christ saves us in all those ways. He sets us aside for safe-keeping. I heard it put this way once: Law condemns even the best; grace saves even the worst. So, "Do not fear, for I have redeemed you; I have called you by name; you are Mine!"(Isaiah 43:1 BSB). He performed the works required to satisfy God so that we don't need to. He came "to seek and to save that which was lost" (Luke 19:10 NASB)—us. The grace of God through Christ offers salvation to all people. Law demands, but grace imparts, and where sin abounds, grace over abounds (Romans 5). Even man's best efforts cannot prevent him from receiving the wages of sin, which is death. Jesus' final act as man conquered the last enemy, death. Jesus gave His life in order to open the door for us to receive eternal life. Salvation "has now been revealed through the appearing of our Savior, Christ Jesus, who has destroyed death and has brought life and immortality to light through the gospel" (2 Timothy 1:10). Through Christ, we are free from the stain of sin and the sting of death.

God's chosen people, the Israelites, had become enslaved and oppressed by the Egyptians. God said, "I have surely seen the affliction of My people who are in Egypt...I am aware of their sufferings. So, I have come down to deliver them from the power of the Egyptians, and to bring them up from that land to a good and spacious land, to a land flowing with milk and honey" (Exodus 3:7-8 NASB). They were liberated by God's mighty hand through Moses. But slavery is not just a part of history; it is alive and well even today. Anything can hold a man captive, and that is what makes him a slave. There's a line from Bob Marley's "Redemption Song" that goes like this: "Emancipate yourselves from mental slavery."[3] Sometimes, we may need to be freed from our own thoughts. The power of Christ is a mighty weapon, used to "knock down the strongholds of human reasoning...destroy every proud obstacle...and capture rebellious thoughts"(2 Corinthians 10:4,5 NLT).

However, redemption in Jesus is much more than just freedom. It is a restoration of that which He did not take. He promises to give back the years that the locusts have eaten. He restores our health and even our very soul. He gives us beauty for ashes and joy for mourning. Just as God saw the oppression of his people, Jesus Christ sees every injustice and is prepared to act on our behalf. Every unfair treatment we endure is an opportunity to receive a greater blessing from Him because He always gives back more than was lost. Remember that Job lost everything, but "the Lord restored the fortunes of Job...and the Lord increased all that Job had two-fold" (Job 42:10 NASB).

Jesus came to restore that which He did not take.

After my divorce, my children went to live with their dad. Two years later, he decided to move a thousand miles away without telling me. That was a terrible loss for me. When I finally found them, I traveled long distance as much as possible for the first couple of years in order to see them. They would move sporadically and never attempted to keep in touch. Presently, I haven't seen my children in three years and the only contact I have with them is a postal box, to which I send cards and cookies. Sadly, they do not respond. It is an unfair and devastating circumstance, for all of us. However, God has graced me with a wonderful step-son, two beautiful step-daughters, and four phenomenal grandchildren. (All of whom appreciate my cookies by the way!) Although nothing can ever replace my own children, I have come to believe that His grace really is sufficient for me and have learned to echo the words of Job, "But as for me, I know that my *Redeemer* lives..."(Job 19:25 NLT).

A HIGHER LOVE

The word "lord" is found over 6,000 times in the Bible. We should be familiar with what one is. Definitively, a "lord" is simply someone who has authority, control or power over others, i.e. master, chief or ruler. The United Kingdom's Parliament, its governmental entity, has a division that is called The House of Lords. They are responsible for reviewing all bills and act as the country's Supreme Court. However, their jurisdiction and ability to pass legislation is minimal. Jesus' lordship, however, is far superior to any man's, for He is limitless in both power and domain. Jesus reigns eternally and has dominion over all things, both in heaven and on earth. In fact, "On his robe and on his thigh, he has this name written: *King of kings* and *Lord of lords*" (Revelation 19:16). He alone was granted that distinct authority by God, who "highly exalted Him, and bestowed on Him the name which is above every name, so that at the name of Jesus every knee will bow, of those who are in heaven and on earth and under the earth, and that every tongue will confess that Jesus Christ is Lord, to the glory of God the Father" (Philippians 2:9-11 NASB). Even prideful men who resist His authority will eventually have to acknowledge Him as Lord.

Jesus is limitless in both power and domain.

Traditionally, becoming a lord was a matter of birth. Only royalty was privileged enough to receive that honor. As the only begotten *Son of God*, Jesus is royalty and "Through him all things were made; without him nothing was made that has been made" (John 1:3). Proverbs describes wisdom personified as being with God during all of creation: "Then I was a skilled craftsman at His side, filled with His delight day by day, rejoicing always in His presence. I was rejoicing in His whole world, delighting together in the sons of men" (Proverbs 8:30-31 BSB). How suitable it was for God to send his heavenly Son to be the earthly son of a carpenter!

When my father died, I felt robbed of "family," and when my mother found another love and began a new life with him and his children, I felt robbed of my childhood home. As a young adult, I had hoped that I would always have a place to come "home" to, but that was not my reality. Although I am very happy for my mother and I genuinely love my step-dad, I carry a bit of sadness about what was lost. However, I have come to know that God causes all things to work together for good to those who love Him. There exists a heavenly home, which God inhabits, and His only son is "at the right hand of the throne of God" (Hebrews 12:2). God has spoken to us though his Son, "whom He appointed the heir of all things, and through whom also he made the universe" (Hebrews 1:2). Although God exists eternally, He has handed all things over to Jesus Christ. This point is very important to grasp. Jesus is both a son to God, and a father to us. So then, "if we are children, then we are heirs—heirs of God and co-heirs with Christ..." (Romans 8:17). Jesus is delighted to share with us all that He has received from His father, saying, "Come, you who are blessed of My Father, inherit the kingdom prepared for you from the foundation of the world" (Matthew 25:34 NASB). He knows that "Both the one who makes people holy, and those who are made holy are of the same family. So, Jesus is not ashamed to call them brothers and sisters" (Hebrews 2:11).

Many of my girl-friends had older brothers that watched out for their little sisters, so I always wished that I had one, too. Jesus Christ is referred to as being the firstborn among many brethren(Romans 8:29) so, technically that makes Jesus my older brother. At least that's how I like to see it. He is our "big brother" and He is protective of us. Having inherited a spiritual family of countless members and an eternal home gives me a sense of belonging which is of far greater value than anything on this earth. Anything I thought I lost, He has more than replaced.

A NAME ABOVE ALL NAMES

God has given Jesus a name above every name and there is power in it. We receive forgiveness by confessing faith *in His name.* We are both justified and sanctified by being baptized *in His name.* We gain access to God by praying *in His name.* We receive salvation by calling upon His name, for "everyone who calls on the name of the Lord will be saved" (Romans 10:13). His name has the power to raise the dead, make the lame walk, and heal all types of disease. In His name, you can "Stretch out your hand to heal and perform signs and wonders through the name of your holy servant Jesus"(Acts 4:30).

Even demons shudder at the name of Jesus. When I was about fifteen years old, my friend and I went to a Haunted House. After we bought our tickets, we headed down a long dark corridor. I heard slight echoes of screams and saw a strobe light flashing up ahead. Then, suddenly, a door opened behind me and "Freddy Krueger" jumped out and started to chase me. My friend outran me, and I tripped and fell to the ground. I was frozen with fear as this dreadful character loomed over me, running his handful of knives through my hair. I screamed, "JESUS!" Immediately the guy stopped and just ran away. I got up and ran until I reached the padded door at the exit, very much thankful to be out. Not being quite mature enough to completely explain what had happened, I mostly kept it to myself. But I always knew that there was something powerful about the name of Jesus. His name is "a strong tower; the righteous run to it and are safe." (Proverbs 18:10 BSB). Even from Freddy Krueger.

There are a few other points about Jesus that make him especially precious to me. He heals the brokenhearted and binds up their wounds (Psalm 147:3). He is the great *physician* and healer. No one can heal like Jesus. He is "the stone which the builders rejected" (Psalm 118:22 NASB). He is now the *chief cornerstone* and the very foundation of my faith. Jesus didn't possess any of the things in this life that we all strive to acquire, yet He wants to give us the desires of our hearts. He said, "I have come that they may have life, and have it abundantly" (John 10:10 BLB). He is the grand supplier. In Him, I have found the key to *everything* in Heaven and on Earth.

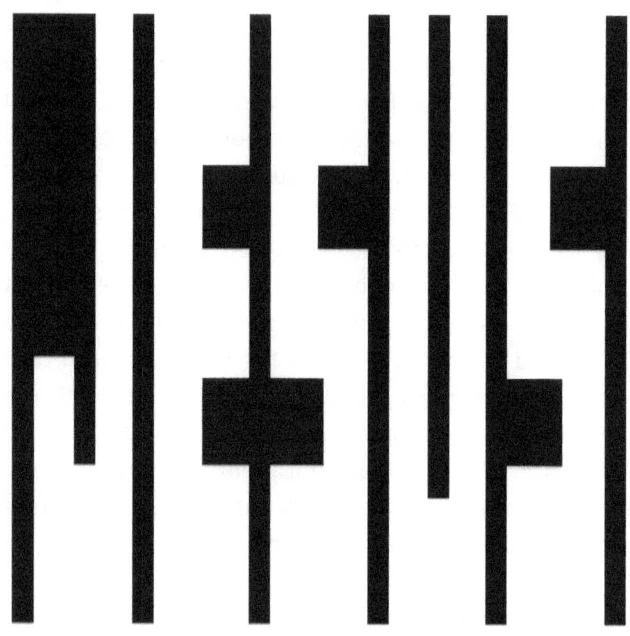

"There was nothing beautiful or majestic
about his appearance,
nothing to attract us to him.
He was despised and rejected—
a man of sorrows, acquainted with deepest
grief.
We turned our backs on him and looked the
other way.
He was despised, and we did not care.
Yet it was our weaknesses he carried;
it was our sorrows that weighed him down.
And we thought his troubles were a
punishment from God,
a punishment for his own sins!
But he was pierced for our rebellion,
crushed for our sins.
He was beaten so we could be whole.
He was whipped so we could be healed.
All of us, like sheep, have strayed away.
We have left God's paths to follow our own.
Isaiah 53:2-6 (NLT)

For to us a child is born,
to us a son is given,
and the government will be on his shoulders.
And he will be called
Wonderful Counselor, Mighty God,
Everlasting Father, Prince of Peace.
Of the greatness of his government and
peace
there will be no end.
He will reign on David's throne
and over his kingdom,
establishing and upholding it
with justice and righteousness
from that time on and forever.
Isaiah 9:6-7

Word Search

```
W H N P U R N H D X W E X A M P L E N R
D R E H P E H S D O O G H A P M C Y W V
L M D K V G H I G H P R I E S T U C D V
M X D Y S F B R T L T A E N B M E C N X
J J H D K L T J F Y L R F A O B K P N H
R G J L S O N J F K B L I C W I R D H D
S E L E T S N X U V R H S N Y C L Q W P
U G H N X A B S B R E A D O F L I F E I
A L H T H H H K B G O F U T H S I N O Q
W Q N L A B M A L F L A B T I B O U L C
B K N M N F O J A I M R U M K B U B X A
I I E B U N F U H G Y R I L L D C S J F
D V Y A G W H A T S T A X E G D U J F G
L D O M D X Y O Y G R Y A W R H D A Y A
R G J I I K V C A A I B H T T T L U I A
O R F W Y A E T B U F O G S D V H A M J
W R Q P T K D B R A T S G N I N R O M B
E N E D B P I R F T F T W X C I T D H J
H E N D P Q M E O S O X L L T H C D S F
T H E I E U X F N W N A Y T J T A M N V
F F A M B E E I T N E U O C D E T A X Q
O S E V B O M L T M K H P A N R P Q R I
T T W X W W B E C Q R B T M E Q O N G U
H J T Y B C Q P R E L Y B R I O W L A O
G C V L T F F V C V O C M T R N X G G O
I F F P O O R E S M X U J M F S Q M J T
L C M P E X W F N O C J W A U L A Q U X
M G S O M R W H M B I V H D D E T X B H
S J A D C I O X A W M C U N W N I W D L
B P R I N C E O F P E A C E O R L F G C
```

**SON   FATHER   REDEEMER   PRINCEOFPEACE   GOODSHEPHERD   JUDGE
LION   LAMB   LORD   FRIEND   HIGHPRIEST   WAY   TRUTH   LIFE   EXAMPLE
LIGHTOFTHEWORLD   THEWORD   MORNINGSTAR   BREADOFLIFE   RABBI**

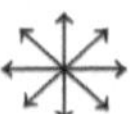

ANSWER ON PAGE V

Chapter 6

I CAN SEE CLEARLY NOW

After long periods of rain, it is always a joy to see the sunshine. When the ground is wet and the water is still dripping from the trees, there is a sense of tranquility that I just love. Observing nature shows me how life really is. It's full of wonder and imagination, sometimes appearing to be something that it is not. It looks much different up-close than from a distance and is often unexpected and unpredictable. Dark clouds can fill our skies, storms may come, and we can even find ourselves living "in a fog." It is during those times when it is most important to be prepared accordingly. The cars we drive have windshield wipers and fog lights. In our homes, we have flashlights, spare batteries, and back-up generators. But what do we have to help us when the *real* storms of life hit us? It's not tucked in a closet somewhere. We can't turn it on or off. We can't even see it. It's God's Holy Spirit. But how do we utilize it? The answer to that question is...by faith. Faith is the *key*. It is our faith that ignites the power of the Holy Spirit.

Keys symbolize security. We use them to unlock our homes and offices, start our cars and lawnmowers, and, sometimes, check our mail at the post office. Keys ensure that only specific people gain access. My husband and I have our own painting and cleaning business, and we often have work that requires entry into a home at a time when the homeowner will not be there. In that case, they give us a key, trusting that their home will be in good hands. But having a key and knowing what to do with it are two different things. When my children were teething, I would give them a set of plastic keys that they loved to chew on. They knew exactly how to use those keys! Knowing how to use a key, as basic as it may seem, is a learned skill. In this day of push button ignitions and remote-control fobs, using a key seems to becoming less common, yet still necessary. If you have ever visited a car dealership, you have probably seen a wall of car keys. You could go over and take your pick. But simply possessing the key would not do you any good. You would also have to know which car it belonged to. Similarly, if we are to use faith properly, we need to understand what it is, how to use it responsibly, and what we are gaining access to by doing so.

Jesus used the word "faith" more than any other word. He possessed the power to heal, but it was a person's faith that caused the healing. He touched their eyes and said, "According to your *faith* let it be done to you" (Matthew 9:29). A woman on the street stretched her hand out to touch the hem of his garment, and when He saw her, he told her, "Daughter, your *faith* has healed you. Go in peace" (Luke 8:48). Faith is defined in the Bible as the assurance of the things we hope for and the proof of things we do not see. Faith convinces us of their reality. In other words, faith perceives as fact that which our senses do not reveal. More simply put, faith says yes, when the world says no.

Faith is viewing life's circumstances from a heavenly perspective.

Abraham believed in God's promise of descendants as "numerous as the stars," even when, naturally speaking, he and Sarah were too old to have children. Scripture says of Abraham: "Without becoming weak in faith he contemplated his own body, now as good as dead since he was about a hundred years old, and the deadness of Sarah's womb" (Romans 4:19 NASB). By faith, Mary believed the angel who told her she was to have a child, even though she had not "had relations with a man" (Luke 1:34 ISV). Faith keeps us in expectation of that which only the Holy Spirit can do. Some things naturally do not seem possible, but spiritually, all things are possible. So, faith is viewing life's circumstances from a heavenly perspective. Paul said it this way: "But a natural man does not accept the things of the Spirit of God, for they are foolishness to him; and he cannot understand them, because they are spiritually appraised" (1 Corinthians 2:14 NASB).

WHAT YOU DON'T KNOW CAN HURT YOU

All five of our human senses can undermine our ability to use faith. Leading a Spirit-led life requires that we train ourselves to maneuver differently in our environment and respond accordingly.

Mastering the skill of walking by faith requires trusting the Holy Spirit and plenty of practice.

If you were flying a plane, and clouds suddenly filled the view out your window, your initial reaction would probably be to panic. That is why one of the things you must master in flight school is "flying blind." The flight simulator takes away your vision, and you must completely rely on your instruments for navigation. A good pilot must learn to trust his instruments, even when he can't trust what he sees. God has given us the greatest instrument of all, the Holy Spirit, who is our helper. Regardless of what we can or cannot see, the Holy Spirit's power is there to guide and direct our steps and helps us to "fix our eyes not on what is seen, but on what is unseen. For what is seen is temporary, but what is unseen is eternal" (2 Corinthians 4:18 BSB). Just like a pilot learning his craft, mastering the skill of walking by faith requires trusting the Holy Spirit and plenty of practice.

Faith guides us in our choices. There are many hidden things in life that we simply do not see. That is why we need direction from the Spirit of God. Jesus said, "But when he, the Spirit of truth, comes, he will guide you into all the truth" (John 16:13).

There is a demand for absolute truth that cannot be acquired by human intellect. In today's market place media, a person has trouble knowing what to believe. We attribute the challenges that come with the mass of media input a phenomenon unique to this era. In reality, however, this is nothing new. The Old Testament shows us that the truth has eluded man from the beginning. In pleading this case, Isaiah cries out to God, "Truth has stumbled in the streets, honesty cannot enter. Truth is nowhere to be found…"(Isaiah 59:14-15). This sentiment is echoed in the New Testament. Even among those who knew Jesus, there were varied opinions or "truths":

> *When Jesus came to the region of Caesarea Philippi, he asked his disciples, "Who do people say the Son of Man is?"*
> *They answered, "Some say you are John the Baptizer, others Elijah, still others Jeremiah or one of the prophets."*
> *He asked them, "But who do you say I am?"*
> *Simon Peter answered, "You are the Messiah, the Son of the living God!"*

Jesus replied, "Simon, son of Jonah, you are blessed! No human revealed this to you, but my Father in heaven revealed it to you."
(Matthew 16:13-16 GWT)

There is no reasoning your way into spiritual truths. The Holy Spirit reveals them to us only through a trusting heart. When the Samaritan woman met Jesus at the well, she responded naturally.

Jesus said to her, "Will you give me a drink?"

The Samaritan woman said to him, "You are a Jew and I am a Samaritan woman. How can you ask me for a drink?" (For Jews do not associate with Samaritans.)

Jesus answered her, "If you knew the gift of God and who it is that asks you for a drink, you would have asked him, and he would have given you living water."

"Sir," the woman said, "you have nothing to draw with and the well is deep. Where can you get this living water? Are you greater than our father Jacob, who gave us the well and drank from it himself, as did also his sons and his livestock?"

Jesus answered, "Everyone who drinks this water will be thirsty again, but whoever drinks the water I give them will never thirst. Indeed, the water I give them will become in them a spring of water welling up to eternal life."

The woman said to him, "Sir, give me this water so that I won't get thirsty and have to keep coming here to draw water."
(John 4:7-15)

He then reveals to her the truth about her own life, and she realizes to whom she is speaking. He goes on to explain to her that people do not need to worship God in a physical place, but that "true worshipers will worship the Father in spirit and in truth. The Father is looking for those who will worship him that way. For God is Spirit, so those who worship him must worship in spirit and in truth" (John 4:23-24 NLT). Jesus reveals the truth of who He is and, in doing so, strengthens her faith.

Skepticism can keep you from walking by faith. Doubting Thomas wouldn't believe that Jesus had been raised from the dead. He wanted proof. Jesus invited him to see and feel His pierced hands. Jesus appeared and said to Thomas, "You believe because you've seen me. Blessed are those who haven't seen me but believe"(John 20:29 GWT). James gives us some rather pointed counsel regarding doubt. He says, "But let him ask in faith, doubting nothing, for the one doubting is like a wave of the sea, being blown and being tossed by the wind. For let that man not suppose that he will receive anything from the Lord. He is a double-minded man, unstable in all his ways" (James 1: 6-8 BLB). An unstable life is insecure and dangerous and is the direct opposite of a spirit-led one.

God works miracles and supplies us the Holy Spirit based upon the *hearing of our faith*, not the doing of our works (Galatians 3:5). As we exercise our faith, it grows stronger, and so does our courage, for "the Spirit God gave us does not make us timid but gives us power, love, and self-discipline" (2 Timothy 1:7). We can courageously face adversity and boldly take leaps of faith, knowing that we have the silent power of Christ within us. Conversely, failure to exercise faith in God leaves us powerless.

Faith requires an all-in commitment. There can be no argument, no compromise, no reservations. It is never wise to attempt to "out think" God because even our own ego can prevent us from living a faith-filled life and keep us from our destination. The following story paints this picture very accurately:

Although unauthenticated, this is the transcript of an ACTUAL radio conversation of a US naval ship with Canadian authorities off the coast of Newfoundland in October 1995:

Americans: Please divert your course 15 degrees to the North to avoid collision.

Canadians: Recommend you divert your course 15 degrees to the South to avoid collision.

Americans: This is the Captain of a US Navy ship. I say again, divert your course.

Canadians: No. I say again, you divert your course.

Americans: This is the aircraft carrier USS Lincoln, the second largest ship in the United States' Atlantic fleet. We are accompanied by three destroyers, three cruisers, and numerous support vessels. I demand that you change your course 15 degrees North. That's one five degrees North, or counter-measures will be undertaken to ensure the safety of this ship.

Canadians: Sir, this is a lighthouse. Your call.

Radio conversation released by the Chief of Naval Operations October 10, 1995[1]

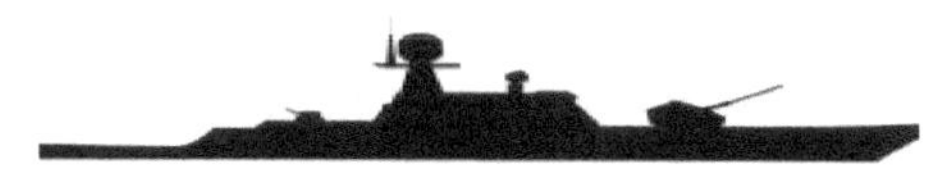

IT'S BLACK OR WHITE

Even with Jesus as an ever-present companion, people of His day had difficulty deciphering the difference between the realm of spiritual truth and physical life. Some of His followers thought Jesus was to become their *earthly* King, even though He had said repeatedly that His Kingdom was not of this world. Some of His disciples argued over who would be the greatest among them when He came to power, when Jesus clearly taught that the least would be greatest in His kingdom. Jesus miraculously fed thousands by multiplying a few loaves of bread, yet his disciples worried about not having any bread. Jesus responded to them saying, "Having eyes, do you not see? And having ears, do you not hear? And do you not remember?" (Mark 8:18 BSB). He was pointing out that there is a difference in seeing versus perceiving and hearing versus understanding. Thankfully, the Holy Spirit helps us in our weakness, knowing full well we are only human. He is working on our behalf even when we may not see it: "In the same way...we do not know what we ought to pray for, but the Spirit himself intercedes for us through wordless groans" (Romans 8:26). That is a cherished gift.

We must understand that we are at war—not with each other—but with the supernatural. In Paul's words, "...our struggle is not against flesh and blood, but against the rulers, against the authorities, against the powers of this dark world and against the spiritual forces of evil in the heavenly realms" (Ephesians 6:12). Though unseen, this war is real, and we all are affected by the battles taking place. Just as there is a spiritual realm, there exists a Heaven, which is the Kingdom of God. We become witnesses of that Kingdom by power of the Spirit. During a conversation with Nicodemus, one of the Pharisees, Jesus tells him that, unless a man be born again, he cannot see the Kingdom of God. Nicodemus reasons that no man can re-enter his mother's womb, but Jesus continues saying, "...no one can enter the kingdom of God unless they are born of water and the Spirit. Flesh gives birth to flesh, but the Spirit gives birth to spirit.

You should not be surprised at my saying, 'You must be born again.' The wind blows wherever it pleases. You hear its sound, but you cannot tell where it comes from or where it is going. So it is with everyone born of the Spirit" (John 3:5-8). This concept was difficult for Nicodemus to understand, as it is with some of us.

Unless a man be born again, he cannot see the Kingdom of God.

One way to aid our comprehension is to look at water baptism as symbolic of being born again. We are called to be baptized and to receive the gift of the Holy Spirit (Acts 2:38). Even Jesus was baptized at the start of His ministry. Paul writes, "Therefore we have been buried with Him through baptism into death, so that as Christ was raised from the dead through the glory of the Father, so we too might walk in newness of life" (Romans 6:4 NASB). We have been given a natural body, which is of the earth, like Adam. Then we are given a spiritual one, which is of heaven, like Jesus. There is a liberty that comes with being born again: "Now the Lord is the Spirit, and where the Spirit of the Lord is, there is freedom" (2 Corinthians 3:17). That freedom is not so that we may do our own will, but rather that we will no longer be slaves to the law of sin and death. We have become recipients of God's grace. Peter wrote it this way: "for you have been born again not of seed which is perishable but imperishable, that is, through the living and enduring word of God"(1 Peter 1:23 NASB).

Because we are both flesh and spirit and there is a struggle between the invisible forces of good and evil, we feel the tension. Galatians 5:17 tells us, "For the flesh desires what is contrary to the Spirit, and the Spirit what is contrary to the flesh.

They are in conflict with each other so that you are not to do whatever you want." There is a simple Cherokee Legend about a grandfather who wanted to share some life wisdom with his grandson. "A fight is going on inside me," he said to the boy. "It is a terrible fight, and it is between two wolves. One is evil—he is anger, envy, greed, arrogance, self-pity, self-doubt, guilt, resentment, inferiority, lies, and ego. The other is good—he is joy, love, hope, serenity, humility, kindness, compassion, empathy, generosity, truth and faith. This same fight is going on inside you and inside every other person, too." The grandson thought about it for a minute and then asked his grandfather, "Which wolf will win?" The old chief simply replied, "The one you feed." We must decide whether we will feed our "flesh," which is full of flaws or our "spirit" which is of God. Whichever one we nurture will determine how the conflict is resolved.

I often sing to myself in my head. It helps me keep my mind focused on spiritual things. There is a simple little song that speaks louder to me than a million words. It goes like this:

> *O be careful little eyes what you see,*
> *O be careful little eyes what you see*
> *For the Father up above*
> *He's looking down in love,*
> *So, be careful little eyes what you see.*[2]

Its multiple verses go on in the same way, replacing "eyes" with, ears, tongue, hands, feet, and heart. To me, it's a great reminder that God loves me and that being careful helps me to "feed" the right "wolf."

The works of our corruptible physical nature are these: illicit sex, perversion, promiscuity, idolatry, drug use, hatred, rivalry, jealousy, angry outbursts, selfish ambition, conflict, factions, envy, drunkenness, wild partying, and similar things. Those all feed the evil wolf. The fruit of the incorruptible Spirit is love, joy, peace, patience, kindness, goodness, faithfulness, gentleness, and self-control. These all feed the good wolf. These wolves cannot feed themselves, and one must dominate. We are admonished to "rid [ourselves] of all such things as these: anger, rage, malice, slander, and filthy language from your lips....clothe [ourselves] with compassion, kindness, humility, gentleness, and patience" (Colossians 3:8,12). Being governed by the Spirit is a deliberate decision to step out in faith. It leads to a fruitful life and peace and prevents us from pleasing our flesh. The Spirit of God renews our hearts and minds and empowers our obedience: "Since we live by the Spirit, let us keep in step with the Spirit" (Galatians 5:25). The phrase here, *in step*, indicates walking in a row or within a rank, just as a soldier does. That means not marching to the beat of our own drum, for doing so would, in fact, make us rebels. We would be the people described in Ezekiel: "They have eyes to see but do not see, and ears to hear but do not hear, for they are a rebellious house" (Ezekiel 12:2). I know this from personal experience. Living my life in rebellion to God led to unnecessary pain and loss.

There is no gray area when it comes to living a Spirit-led life.

One of the gravest mistakes we can make is to believe that we can occupy neutral ground in trying to live for God. There is no light in darkness, no harmony between Christ and the devil, and no grace under law. There is no compromising with the world, for the world is the enemy of the Kingdom of Heaven. This may seem to be a bit harsh, but God has only given us two choices—the narrow gate, which leads to life, or the broad gate, which leads to destruction (Matthew 7:13-14) God told the Israelites:

Today I have given you the choice between life and death, between blessings and curses. Now I call on heaven and earth to witness the choice you make. Oh, that you would choose life, so that you and your descendants might live! You can make this choice by loving the Lord your God, obeying him, and committing yourself firmly to him. This is the key to your life. (Deuteronomy 30:19-20 NLT)

There is no gray area when it comes to living a Spirit-led life. Time does not stop to wait for us to decide which way to go; life just goes on. We either choose to catch the wave of the spirit, or we are left stagnating. Just as a surfer may choose to wait for the perfect wave, we might like to think that we can pick and choose which things to be faithful in. The truth is that the "perfect wave" may never come, and the only way to score is to risk going all in. In other words, take advantage of every opportunity to exercise your faith, and you will succeed in living a Spirit-led life. The book of Revelation goes on to say, "I know your deeds; you are neither cold nor hot. How I wish you were one or the other! So, because you are lukewarm—neither hot nor cold —I'm about to vomit you out of My mouth" (Revelation 3:15-16 BSB). Walking according to the Spirit can be uncomfortable at first, but with training and practice, it becomes glorious. For the "mystery that has been hidden and that God destined for our glory before time began...no human mind has conceived...these are the things God has revealed to us by his Spirit. The Spirit searches all things, even the deep things of God" (1 Corinthians 2:7-10).

The ocean is deep and vast and contains some very unique and intriguing things. Only a select few have been able to venture to its deepest parts. How much greater is the depth of God's wisdom and power that man cannot even begin to measure it. Be prepared to be amazed.

Put Your Money Where Your Mouth Is

Exercising faith in God means that our actions line up with our words. God's amazing grace, truth, and faithfulness towards us should cause us to respond in confidence. If you were to travel to a foreign country whose monetary system was different from yours, you would need to exchange your currency for theirs. Similarly, faith can be likened to the currency which operates the Kingdom of God. So, investing in the Kingdom of Heaven requires us to have and use faith. Paul said, "It is impossible to please God without faith. Anyone who wants to come to him must believe that God exists and that he rewards those who sincerely seek him" (Hebrews 11:6 NLT).

Charles Blondin, a French acrobat, was made famous in the United States for tightrope walking across Niagara Falls. It was the summer of 1859, and Charles had already made headlines for his antics as an acrobat. While up on the rope without a net, he would walk across backwards, run, lie down, hang from one arm or stop midway in order to sip wine from a bottle he had hoisted up from a boat below. He crossed from side to side, first carrying a balancing pole, then blindfolding himself by covering his head with a burlap sack. He crossed as many ways as he think up: at night by locomotive lights, while wearing shackles, carrying people, tables, chairs and even a stove (which he would light and use to cook an omelet). Crowds of thousands would flock to watch him. They couldn't wait to see what he would do next. He crossed Niagara Falls 300 times during his life. You might say that he was a little crazy, but he must have had faith in some capacity.

One of the most memorable moments of his performances was when he traversed the rope pushing a wheelbarrow. Then he put on his blindfold. As was usual, he asked the crowd if they thought he could do it. They shouted, "Yes!" Then he asked them if they thought he could do it with a person inside the barrow. Once again, they shouted, enthusiastically, "Yes!" Then he asked them who would volunteer to ride. A hush fell over the crowd. Of course, no one volunteered. He had proven he could do it time and time again, but the crowd was not willing to act upon what they claimed to believe. In the same way, when we say that we trust God with our lives, how do we show it? James said, "Faith by itself, if it is not accompanied by action, is dead" (James 2:17). Words are words, and promises are promises. Only action is reality. Walking by faith and not by sight requires us to "put our money where our mouth is."

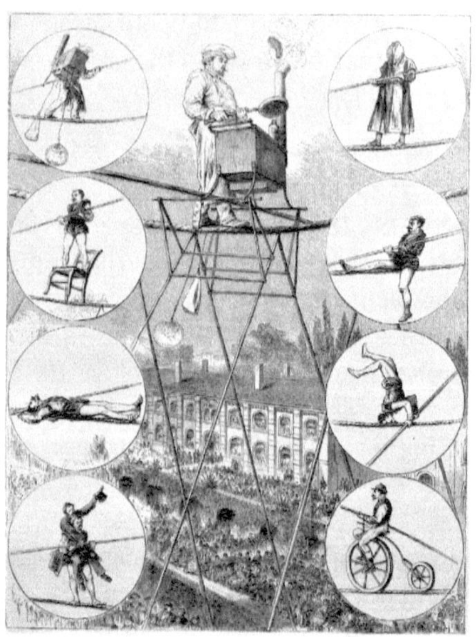

Eye on the Finish Line

All the riches, wisdom, and glory of this world amount to nothing in comparison to the Kingdom of God. Scholars estimate that King Solomon's net worth, in today's value, would be at two trillion dollars, making him the richest king to ever have lived. Even the land of his kingdom was extremely rich, providing twenty-five tons of gold each year from its mines. He acquired distant fame and many women. Seemingly, he had the grandest life a man could ever have, yet he held this rather unconventional truth: "The day of one's death is better than the day of one's birth" (Ecclesiastes 7:1 NASB). Solomon was the wisest king who ever lived, and he understood the temporal nature of this life. It is the eternal life that only comes after this earthly one that is the real treasure. Jesus said that there are many rooms in His Father's house, and that He is going to prepare a place for us, returning to bring us back to live with Him (John 14:2-3). It is by faith that we live and we wait.

Now we live with great expectation, and we have a priceless inheritance— an inheritance that is kept in heaven for you, pure and undefiled, beyond the reach of change and decay. And through your faith, God is protecting you by his power until you receive this salvation, which is ready to be revealed on the last day for all to see. So be truly glad. (1 Peter 1:3-6 NLT)

While we confidently and joyfully look forward to sharing God's glory, we presently live according to the promise that the same Spirit who raised Jesus from the dead lives in us. We live and exist only in Him (Acts 17:28). When problems and trials come our way, we can "rejoice, too...for we know that they help us develop endurance. And endurance develops strength of character, and character strengthens our confident hope of salvation. And this hope will not lead to disappointment" (Romans 5:3-5 NLT). I have come to understand that there are many "believers" who simply need to know that they are not alone. We all need each other. We especially need the power of the Holy Spirit for strength, comfort, and direction. We are supported by those who have come before us. We have a race to run and one life in which to run it.

> *Therefore, since we are surrounded by such a great cloud of witnesses, let us throw off everything that hinders and the sin that so easily entangles. And let us run with perseverance the race marked out for us.*
>
> *(Hebrews 12:1)*

Chapter 7

HOW DOES YOUR GARDEN GROW?

I really enjoy gardening—planting flowers, feeling the soil in my hands, watching things grow, and picking vegetables fresh from the vine. I even took some horticulture classes at the local college and got a job managing a greenhouse. By far, that was one of the most enjoyable jobs I ever had. As a greenhouse, we not only grew plants but served as consultants for landscape design and plant selection. I met many customers who wanted to have great lawns and productive gardens, but it was often challenging to find just the right layout that suited them. Most of us enjoy expressing ourselves in our own way, and our lawns and gardens are no exception. The size, type, and purpose vary from house to house, but there are some uniform elements that are necessary for every garden's success. The foundation should be made of well-drained soil, and plants need to be rooted at the proper depth and distance from one another. Establishing healthy plants that bloom and thrive requires certain nutrients, sunshine, and rain. Similarly, our heart needs to be cultivated in order to allow the word of God to take root. We need the sunshine of our Father's love and the rain of the Holy Spirit to make our faith grow. In addition, there are definitely essential *nutrients* for the Spirit-led life that make our surrendering to God a success. When established properly, our life will reflect what is spoken of in Psalms 1:3, "He will be like a tree firmly planted by streams of water, which yields its fruit in its season and its leaf does not wither; and in whatever he does, he prospers"(NASB) But just like a garden's needs change with the seasons, our needs may as well. So, it is important to regularly tend our "garden" and pay attention to what may be required.

BIBLE STUDY

Bible study is crucial to a healthy spiritual life. Never lose the necessity of having God as your teacher because you can never reach perfect understanding on your own. Reading a chapter, or —worse—a single verse only one time does not give me discernment. I have found that spiritual truths are most often revealed in numerous passages and through repetition. A few years ago, I completed a course through Notre Dame University that taught me a practice called Lectio Divina, which literally means "divine reading." This method allows you to familiarize yourself with a select chapter or group of scriptures within the Bible and get the most value from your reading. After I select the scriptures, I read them slowly and think on the entire passage. Then I reread the same passage again. Only this time, I do so prayerfully, asking God to point out what there is to learn from it. As I read, I try to recognize what stands out. Then, I read the passage one last time, taking simple notes along the way. Incorporating that practice into my study has broadened my insight on much of scripture and never fails to impress me.

When reading the Bible, I keep this thought in mind: Text without context is simply pretext. Verses in and of themselves may be easy to remember, but it is more important that we understand the circumstances upon which the verse was written. For example: Proverbs 5:18 says, "...may you rejoice in the wife of your youth." Malachi 2:14 says, "The Lord is the witness between you and the wife of your youth. You have been unfaithful to her..." My ex-husband used those words to justify his decision to leave me and return to his first girlfriend. He actually believed that God was telling him to do so! I was so shocked, and ignorant at the time, that I didn't know what to think. He had taken the scripture out of context and used it for his own purposes. If you read the entire chapter of Proverbs 5, you would soon realize that it is, in fact, a warning *against* adultery. In Malachi, God is referencing the fact that the nation of Judah had forsaken Him by marrying women who worship other gods. It is a plea to return to God and an admonishment *against* divorce. Reading a scripture out of context leads to misinterpretation and can be dangerous for yourself and others.

The Bereans were a group of men noted in the Bible for their way of studying the holy writings. Acts says of them: "Now the Bereans were more noble-minded than the Thessalonians, for they received the message with great eagerness and examined the Scriptures every day to see if these teachings were true"(Acts 17:11 BSB). They were not content to just read the scriptures once and be done; they *studied daily.* Studying the Bible requires more than merely reading the words at face value. Rich truths are embedded within its pages and are often developed over time. That is what I have had to learn. Developing a habit of daily Bible reading has been a learning experience, to say the least. Inspired by God, the Bible was written by 66 different authors over a period of 1500 years or more. It amazes me how all the books relate to one another, often explaining timeless truths, yet all pointing to the same Savior. Saint Augustine expressed it this way: The New Testament is in the Old Testament concealed, and the Old Testament is in the New Testament revealed. There are so many ways to read the Bible that it is difficult for me to recommend just one. The point I want to make clear is that regular study, in whatever capacity, will only help you. We are reminded in 2 Timothy 3:16 that, "all Scripture is God-breathed and is useful for instruction, for conviction, for correction, and for training in righteousness"(BSB).

WORSHIP

Simply attending a church service is good to incorporate into our spiritual life, but true worship of God entails much more. For me, it combines prayer, music, and meditation into a lifestyle of reverence. This is what really strengthens my trust in God, which is the foundation of my life.

Prayer

If I had to pick which of these components was the single most important, by far, this would be the one. There are literally thousands of books written solely on the value of prayer. The Bible tells us to "Pray without ceasing" (1 Thessalonians 5:17 KJV). That means that prayer is a state of being—not an isolated act. It is also as diverse as humanity. It can be done whispering or crying aloud, standing with arms raised or on your knees with folded hands and bowed head, through tears of sorrow or through laughter. It may be standing in a crowd, out on a public street or it may be in the privacy of your own prayer closet. Jesus set the perfect example in this regard. He prayed alone, with others and for others. He prayed short prayers and prayers that lasted all night. He maintained a constant communication with His Father during every moment of His life.

There is no greater feeling than to know that your Maker hears your every word, even if the "words" are silent. Throughout the Bible, we see the prayers of God's faithful ones. Daniel's prayer life is one such example for us. Even those who were not of his faith knew of his faithfulness in praying to God, and they used it to have him thrown into the lion's den. However, he did not allow his circumstances to deter him from praying, and God's angels faithfully rescued him from the mouths of the lions. It is prayer that builds my relationship with God. He is my constant companion, and I long to hear His voice, as Elijah did. Elijah was feeling alone and afraid, and he went up to a mountain where he prayed. A powerful wind came and tore rocks off the mountain, but the Lord was not in the wind. Then a terrible earthquake struck, but the Lord was not in the earthquake either. Then came a fire, but again, the Lord was not in the fire. But after that fire came a "still, small voice. When Elijah heard it, he wrapped his face in his cloak and went out and stood at the entrance of the cave. And a voice said, 'What are you doing here, Elijah?'" (1 Kings 19:13 NLT). That still small voice whispers to us today. It is the comforting sound of our Creator, beckoning us to just be with Him. That is what prayer is to me: the chance to just be still, removed from any distractions, and simply listen for His voice. It is the greatest opportunity to be in quiet connection with God.

Music

Music is a powerful tool of persuasion. About five years ago, I started listening to Christian music on a national radio station, K-LOVE. I took their thirty-day challenge, which was to only listen to Christian music for thirty days. It didn't even take the thirty days before I could feel the difference in my mental and emotional state. I became keenly aware of the negative influence that secular music had on me, so I decided to stop listening to it, *period*.

A Japanese pseudo-scientist by the name Masaru Emoto is known for his experiments dealing with how water is affected by music, words, and emotions. One study highlights musical impressions. Distilled water vials were individually exposed to various types of music: classical, opera, heavy rock etc. As the water "listened" to the music, it was quickly frozen, in order to reveal the individual water crystals. The water that had been exposed to classical music developed the most beautiful and ornate structures, like snowflakes. The crystals that were formed by the water exposed to heavy rock were nearly unrecognizable, chaotic and held no structure. His laboratory performed further studies using words and tone as well, yielding the same results.[1]

The average human body is 50-65% water, so is it any wonder that we would be affected by music as well? The sounds we are exposed to affect us both physically and spiritually. Just as we know that junk food is unhealthy, we know that healthy food makes us look and feel better. Similarly, "feeding" on the music of the world causes us to reflect destructive behavior and emotions while incorporating Godly music into our "diet" gives us nourishment and causes us to feel and act in a more wholesome way. Much of the popular music broadcast these days contains graphic lyrics about sex and violence. It's no wonder that our world is full of the same.

Just as a picture "paints a thousand words," the right song can speak more than just words. Music brings us comfort, helps us to heal, and can even make us rejoice. We all have emotions that we struggle with. For me, it is the feeling of inadequacy. When I start to feel that way, I listen to a song written by Anthony Brown called "Worth," and it reminds me that my value lies in Christ and that Jesus died just for me. We are told in Colossians 3:16 to "let the message of Christ dwell among [us] richly as [we] teach and admonish one another with all wisdom through psalms, hymns, and songs from the spirit, singing to God with gratitude in [our] hearts." This is more than a suggestion; it is a command. Furthermore, praising God in song produces joy—which is our strength.

Meditation

What we spend our time thinking about dominates our emotions and behavior. It makes us who we are. James Allen addresses this same idea in his book As a Man Thinketh, which begins with these lines:

Mind is the Master power that molds and makes,
And Man is Mind, and evermore he takes
The tool of Thought...
And shaping what he wills,

Brings forth a thousand joys, a thousand ills:
He thinks in secret, and it comes to pass:
Environment is but his looking-glass.[2]

Whether we would like to admit it or not, our own thought-world holds the key to every condition, good or bad, that comes into our life. Every thought always precedes action. Proverbs 23:7 says regarding man: "For as he thinketh in his heart, so is he"(KJV).

Most of us have a morning routine, but how many of us take advantage of it being the best time to get our thinking straight? Personally, I like my cup of coffee and the calm of the morning. I have discovered that taking the opportunity to spend that quiet time, by myself with God sets me on a course of grace for the day. Thinking about His greatness, the blessings He has given me or just appreciating nature strengthens my resolve to live out my life in a spiritual way. Lacking that special time in the morning or overthinking my plan for the day negatively impacts the rest of my day. I often find a scripture to keep in my mind throughout the day. It not only keeps my mind set on the things of God, but I find that I have gained greater insight by the end of the day. Paul put it this way: "Finally, brothers and sisters, whatever is true, whatever is noble, whatever is right, whatever is pure, whatever is lovely, whatever is admirable - if anything is excellent or praiseworthy - think about such things" (Philippians 4:8). You can never go wrong thinking good thoughts.

FRIENDS

Real friends are a treasure in this life. The Navi people from the movie Avatar, have a keen sense as to how to treat one another in love. Neytiri and Jake become intimate friends and, according to Navi tradition, greet each other by saying, "I see you."[3] They are not speaking of a literal sight; they are acknowledging the other person's divine nature. That is what true friends do. They see beyond the barriers of social or cultural identity. We are all in this life together so we should learn to share our gifts with others and appreciate the gifts others must share. In the book of Luke, Jesus reminds us to "Give, and it will be given to you. They will pour into your lap a good measure, pressed down, shaken together, and running over. For by your standard of measure it will be measured to you in return" (Luke 6:38 NASB).

Some well rounded advice in this regard is this: Find a friend ahead of you to mentor you, have a friend alongside you to share common ground with, and help others by being a friend to one behind you. That is how the cycle of giving and receiving works. Some people have too many friends, and some don't have enough. Personally, I prefer to think about the quality of friends, rather than the quantity. My best and most treasured friend is my husband, and as such, he respects and honors me as I am. Having him as a trustworthy companion gives me the love and acceptance I need to thrive spiritually. I had a best friend growing up with whom I would spend countless hours. After a few days, we would inevitably start to bicker, and my mother would suggest that we "take a break" from each other. After a day or two, we would be right back to being the two little girls who loved to just hang out. Similarly, because we cannot get away from ourselves, we can end up being our own worst enemy. No one can influence you as effectively as yourself. So, give yourself helpful advice. Forgive yourself when you mess up. Be patient with yourself. Remind yourself that you are deeply loved. Learn to be your own best friend.

HUMILITY

Being humbled can happen suddenly; remaining humble takes practice. Every day we make decisions. The first and most important one is to let go of our ego and seek God's will in our lives. Self-ambition, self-will, self-promotion, and self-gratification are all enemies to our ability to live for God. We must strive to cultivate humility. Humility is not a weakness, as some may say. Quite the contrary. It requires us to toughen up. Most of us, in our nature, want to "go with the flow." We prefer the easy way and like to assume we know things. Humility is essentially the opposite. It is uncomfortable and requires us to follow someone else's direction. C. S. Lewis said that the truly humble man "will not be thinking about humility: he will not be thinking about himself at all."[4] Sometimes it takes great strength to subdue our own soul, but keeping these few points in mind helps me to remain humble:

- Remember how far God has brought you.
- You are a citizen of heaven and, therefore, God is your ruler.
- God knows your desires and flaws, so He knows what is best for you.

God asks us to do what is right, to love mercy, and to walk humbly with Him. That is an open invitation to walk with grace and the opportunity of a lifetime. Walking with God is exactly what Adam lost in Eden, so to know that we can do so again is a treasure worth humbling ourselves for.

COURAGE

Courage is an abstract quality and one that is difficult to explain. I love how C.S. Lewis defines it. He said, "Courage is not simply one of the virtues, but the form of every virtue at its testing point."[5] Anything that we set out to do, especially if it is new for us, requires boldness on our part. Imagine being the first to cross the ocean or go into space. It took courage—moving beyond fear. To me, willingness is the first and most important step to accomplishing anything in life.

There was a book I read back in grade school titled The Red Badge of Courage. The story is about a young soldier who wanted to be on the front lines of the army during the Civil War. However, when the fight grew fierce, he ran away. He encountered many fallen comrades along the way and felt guilty for not remaining in the battle. The author, Stephen Crane, wrote this about the soldier, "At times he regarded the wounded soldiers in an envious way. He conceived persons with torn bodies to be peculiarly happy. He wished he, too, had a wound, a red badge of courage."[6] I can truly empathize with that young soldier. I want to be brave, too. There are times when I wish I would have said or done something that would have been considered bold. But fear often held me back. I lacked the courage to do what my heart desired.

I have seen this aspect of my personality play out in one of my favorite hobbies: photography. I take all kinds of pictures, but the reality is that I miss great shots because I hesitate. In my mind, I think I must wait for just the right moment, but I usually end up missing the whole shot. Hesitating in life leads to missing out on opportunities to grow spiritually. Because we confront every situation with God, we have nothing to fear and everything to gain. King Solomon had this to say on the subject:

> *Ship your grain across the sea;*
> *after many days you may receive a return.*
> *Invest in seven ventures, yes, in eight;*
> *you do not know what disaster may come upon*
> *the land.*
> *If clouds are full of water,*
> *they pour rain on the earth.*
> *Whether a tree falls to the south or to the north,*
> *in the place where it falls, there it will lie.*
> *Whoever watches the wind will not plant;*
> *whoever looks at the clouds will not reap.*
> *As you do not know the path of the wind,*
> *or how the body is formed in a mother's womb,*
> *so you cannot understand the work of God,*
> *the Maker of all things.*
> *Sow your seed in the morning,*

and at evening let your hands not be idle,
for you do not know which will succeed,
whether this or that,
or whether both will do equally well.
-Ecclesiastes 11:1-6

Cultivating my trust in God's eternal word, presence, power, protection, and mercy is what keeps me grounded in courage.

DETERMINATION

During my stay at the emotional recovery center, I met with one of the psychiatrists there. During our meeting, I told him about all the things that were going wrong in my life and how hurt, confused and angry I felt. He told me that I had no problems—just decisions to make. At the time, I was offended because I felt that I had too many problems to even count. But I soon realized that he was absolutely right. My only problem was my inability to decide to change and my lack of fortitude. I had been spending far too much time deciding not to change, keeping the cycle of insanity going. I was stuck. Blind to the fact that my destiny was in my own hands. Every decision we make has the potential to produce a change if we so choose it. Progress is deciding on a deliberate change. Waiting for things to change is possible, but if it is within our power to change for the good, we should. Ignoring things, just thinking they will change on their own someday, is like playing the lottery. You have one in a twelve million chance of winning big one day, but you can't just sit around waiting for it. You must earn money in the meantime in order to survive.

Just as making a grocery list prior to going to the store helps me shop more efficiently, deciding to follow Jesus prior to going about my day makes my life simpler and more convenient. Being determined to continually progress helps me to actively participate in life instead of just watching it fly by. It also helps me make the best use of my time because I don't waste it contemplating what I could do or couldn't do, but never doing it. Now I decide, and, as Nike claims, "just do it." As Jesus said, "Simply let your 'Yes' be 'Yes,' and your 'No,' 'No.' Anything more comes from the evil one" (Matthew 5:37 BSB). Once we decide to do something, our determination helps us to follow through. There's an old saying that warns against burning bridges, but I would have to disagree when it comes to God. Once we decide to live the surrendered life He has for us, we should live as though there is no possible retreat. Only good days lie ahead.

REST

Have you ever tripped while walking or running? Have you ever failed to see something that was right under your nose? Ever been driving and miss your turn? More than likely it was due to you going too fast or perhaps your speed and focus just weren't lining up. In this high-paced world, it can be challenging to slow down and relax as we go through life. But if we are to live an effective and fruitful life, we must learn to rest. Even crop fields need a season of rest in order to yield a good harvest.

Giving our minds and bodies a break helps us to see clearly and avoid rash behavior.

We often mistake our day of rest as a time to do what we haven't been able to do during our work week. However, that is not what God intended for our Sabbath day. Isaiah 58:13 reminds us to "Keep the Sabbath day holy. Don't pursue your own interests on that day but enjoy the Sabbath and speak of it with delight as the LORD's holy day. Honor the Sabbath in everything you do on that day, and don't follow your own desires or talk idly"(NLT). God created the Sabbath for man, not man for the Sabbath. Our obligation to the Sabbath is to honor God for the rest that He has given us. God wants us to enjoy the Sabbath and take the time to be grateful for the many blessings He gives us each day. I am a busy person by nature, so I always have some project going. It is difficult for me to do "nothing." So, I remind myself that resting is not "nothing," but it is an essential time for reflection and rejuvenation. Sometimes when I am working tirelessly on a project, I reach a point when I just can't seem to figure it out, and I get a little frustrated. If I set it aside for a while and then come back to it, I have a fresh outlook, and I can overcome what was never an obstacle to begin with. Similarly, giving our minds and bodies a break helps us to see clearly and avoid rash behavior.

As busy as Jesus was, He knew the importance of taking a reprieve. He had been working with His disciples and so many people had been coming and going that they hadn't even had a chance to eat. So, He said to them, "Come with me by yourselves to a quiet place and get some rest" (Mark 6:31). What really helps me to give myself time to rest is creating an environment in my home that is inviting and serene. When the laundry list of things I "need" to do is staring at me, it is difficult to relax, so a peaceful home is essential for me. Having said that, setting aside that "to do" list for the time being may be the only way to find the time to rest. Church services can be a good way to honor the Sabbath if it is done with the right heart. I heard a preacher once admonish the congregation regarding being in such a rush to get out of church saying, "If you're worried about the dirty dishes setting in the sink at home, don't worry. They'll still be there when you get there." We should avail ourselves of the time we get to share with each other about the great things God has done and encourage one another to stay fixed on Jesus, not circumstance.

Keeping the Sabbath day was a decision that my husband and I made out of obedience, wanting to do so in order to honor God. My husband is a musician and, as such, played every weekend. It was a difficult decision to quit because of the comfort of having that extra money. However, God saw to it that the money that was lost by not playing music was multiplied through other work that was more rewarding. Honoring the Sabbath is not only refreshing but reaps rewards from God "...then you will take delight in the LORD, and he will make you ride upon the heights of the earth" (Isaiah 58:14 ISV).

Bible study, worship, friends, humility, courage, determination, and rest make up a short list of my daily sustenance. Together they provide a buffet of nutrition for me to choose from. Each day I can take in a well-balanced meal. These are the nutrients that my spiritual garden needs to flourish. Individual circumstances and situations come and go, and so there are certain times when I may need more prayer or cannot rest as much. But the important thing for me is to pay attention so that I don't miss out on any one of them. This list is by no means exhaustive nor a one size fits all. It is important to take the time to figure out your personal needs and adjust accordingly. However, there is one simple thing that can be done each and every day regardless of the season. As you finish dressing for the day, remember to "suit yourself" by putting on the whole Armor of God:

> *Stand firm then, with the belt of truth buckled around your waist, with the breastplate of righteousness in place, and with your feet fitted with the readiness that comes from the gospel of peace. In addition to all this, take up the shield of faith, with which you can extinguish all the flaming arrows of the evil one. Take the helmet of salvation and the sword of the Spirit, which is the word of God.*
> *-Ephesians 5:14-17*

Chapter 8

I NEVER PROMISED YOU A ROSE GARDEN

Coach Miles was my elementary school gymnastics coach. He was a tall, drill sergeant kind-of man who always called you by your last name. When he did, you were expected to respond directly. As my spotter, he would look me square in the eye and say, "I've gotcha. You're in good hands with Miles-state" (like the slogan for Allstate insurance). Knowing he was there to keep me from getting hurt gave me the confidence to do what I was learning to do. As I mastered each new skill, I no longer needed a spotter, but Coach Miles would still be there, watching me. The security he provided gave me the freedom to take a risk, even though I was sometimes afraid. We can have that same secure feeling when we first surrender to God, confident we are in good hands. Because we are learning new life skills, there comes a time when we must exercise our faith independently. That is just a part of growing into spiritual maturity. Don't underestimate the power of your faith, and don't ever take it for granted. Think of it as a check which must be taken to a bank in order to have value and be utilized. Deposit it in every situation of your life; make it a habit. Jesus said that even faith the size of a mustard seed could move mountains. So, use your faith as an investment in your new self.

EVERY ROSE HAS ITS THORN

I beg your pardon. I never promised you a rose garden. Along with the sunshine, there's gotta be a little rain sometime. When you take, you gotta give, so live and let live, or let go. I beg your pardon. I never promised you a rose garden.[1]

Joe South wrote those lyrics many years ago, but they are just as relevant today. We can be tempted to think that because we have surrendered our life to God that it's time to just "breathe easy." But remember that even in the rose garden, there are thorns...and pests. We are embarking on a major rebuild which requires quite a bit of work. Anyone who has ever done any home remodeling can understand the concept. My husband and I bought and remodeled a home that was partially built in 1850. In addition to the expected cleaning and painting, the old house required some extensive repairs. We demolished the entire kitchen, had all new plumbing and fixtures installed, and ran practically all new electrical wires. Unexpected issues arose throughout the whole process, so we learned to address them as they came while waiting patiently for our house to be livable. Similarly, as a born-again child of God, we are undergoing restoration and our internal circuits and processes may need to be reestablished. We are under the tutelage of our Creator, so we are no longer just going through life. We are *growing* through life. And a part of that growing process is suffering "growing pains."

If we want something of real value, we must be willing for it to cost us something. You can't expect a free cup of coffee to taste like a three dollar Starbucks Americano. But what if you couldn't see what you were buying? Would you still be willing to "pay up" beforehand? Not many of us would. The unknown makes us uneasy. It inevitably causes us to venture out of our comfort zone. Although we know that God is trustworthy and that He has nothing but our best welfare in mind, there are times when our future is unforeseen. It is in those moments that our faith and trust in God is tested. Woodrow Wilson once said, "Loyalty means nothing unless it has at its heart the absolute principle of self-sacrifice."[2] Trusting God when we can't see the outcome requires the sacrifice of stretching our faith.

The word *sacrifice* denotes a giving up of something. The problem is that most of us find it difficult to give up anything. A bodybuilder, however, understands well the principle of self-sacrifice. If he is determined to gain muscle mass and strength, he must go through a painful process. When weight is lifted, the muscle literally tears. Then the muscles must rest in order to rebuild and heal. The process is repeated over and over, often for years, until the muscles are the size and strength the body builder desires. Bodybuilding requires dedication and discipline. So, does maintaining our submission to God. No reservations, no retreats, no regrets. Once you have chosen to give your life to God, don't try to take it back. Ecclesiastes 5:5 says "it is better not to make a vow than to make one and not fulfill it." When the going gets tough, the tough get going, so they say. Self-preservation will only lead to mediocrity and weakness. You may be tempted to wade in shallow water where you can see clearly to the bottom. But if you want to catch big fish, you must risk the rough waves of the deep blue ocean. Don't long for life to be easier; long to be better. Don't crave fewer problems; crave more skills.

LIFE IS LIKE A BOX OF CHOCOLATES

Life can be unpredictable, but we can avoid the negative impact of "those little surprises" by having reasonable expectations. Here is my list:

- Don't expect things in life—or yourself for that matter—to be flawless.
- Conflict is a part of this life; accept it.

- We simply cannot go through life
without injury, BUT we heal.

- Life can be unfair and there are times
when you will fail; be resilient.

- Life is in constant motion; remaining
the same is not an option.

When I devoted my life to God by getting baptized, things initially went well. I was going to church regularly, studying the bible, praying and even sharing with others what I was learning. I felt confident about what I was doing and thought that I had essentially been "fixed." I was sure that I was on the "right path" and that it was going to be "smooth sailing" from then on. I was wrong. I soon came to realize that our greatest opposition to success can be our latest victory. Luke describes this condition of man:

> *When an unclean spirit comes out of a man, it passes through arid places seeking rest and does not find it. Then it says, 'I will return to the house I left.' On its return, it finds the house swept clean and put in order. Then it goes and brings seven other spirits, more wicked than itself, and they go in and dwell there. And the final plight of that man is worse than the first. (Luke 11:24-25 BSB)*

Spiritual warfare is real, and I have found that devoting our attention to God inevitably gets the attention of His enemy. Even though we have God's guidance and protection, the enemy doesn't just sit back, admit defeat, and leave us alone. He watches us and waits for his opportunity to confront us. Peter warns us to "Stay alert! Watch out for your great enemy, the devil. He prowls around like a roaring lion, looking for someone to devour" (1 Peter 5:8 NLT). When Jesus was baptized, He was led by the Spirit into the desert for forty days of communion with His Father. When He grew hungry, Satan showed up to tempt him. Although Satan's attempts were unsuccessful, Luke 4:13 tells us that, "When the devil had finished all this tempting, he left him until another opportune time." If Satan thinks he can persuade even the son of God to betray his father, we must not think we are exempt from his attacks.

THE ENEMY FROM WITHIN

Although we may be getting spiritually stronger, we all still have our weaknesses. James 1:14 reminds us that "Temptation comes from our own desires, which entice us and drag us away"(NLT). We may have deeply rooted worldly habits or even have worldly friends who can impede our ability to remain under God's authority. Seek to acknowledge those hindrances and pray for help in letting them go. Breaking a bad habit is something I certainly understand. I used to enjoy smoking even though I knew it wasn't healthy. I had tried to quit but it never really worked long-term. I still *wanted* to smoke, so I always came back to it. Then I began praying to God that He take away my desire to smoke. He answered my prayer, and what used to be so satisfying for me has now become something which repels me. 1 John 2:16 tells us, "For the world offers only a craving for physical pleasure, a craving for everything we see, and pride in our achievements and possessions. These are not from the Father, but are from this world"(NLT). In Philippians, Paul explains that there are enemies to the cross, that "their god is their appetite, they brag about shameful things, and they think only about this life here on earth" (Philippians 3:19 NLT). Be cautious of what the world may be offering you and distance yourself from its influence. John admonishes us, "Don't you realize that friendship with the world makes you an enemy of God? I say it again: If you want to be a friend of the world, you make yourself an enemy of God" (James 4:4 NLT). That is a very bold, but true statement. We are a completely new creation and no part of us is exempt from God's dominion.

Be cautious of what the world may be offering you and distance yourself from its influence.

Resilience. Dozens of movies and songs have been written about it. The term "comeback kid" has been readily used to describe someone who has been knocked down but gets back up, been rejected but rebounds. The idea is somewhat nostalgic. Although the sentiment of not backing down is popular, it is really rooted in man's stubbornness. Stubbornness is contrary to our choice to submit to God. Remnants of our old self tend to be stubborn. They like to remind us they are still there through a simple thought or even an emotion, stemming from our old heart condition. However, those old habits are simply carnal appetite and will interfere with hearing God's voice. Recognize them when they show up and strive to listen beyond them in order to stay tuned in to God. Let him have his way with you. Paul says in Colossians 3:15, "Let the peace of Christ rule in your hearts, since as members of one body you were called to peace. And be thankful."   The Bible refers to our heart as the seed of motivation. It is where we hold our feelings and what causes us to act. Jeremiah 17:9 says, "The heart is more deceitful than all else And is desperately sick; Who can understand it?"(NASB) That being true, then the "follow your heart" mentality of the world is not profitable. That advice only seeks to pull us away from God's plan. It is much wiser to "Delight yourself in the Lord and he will give you the desires of your heart" (Psalm 37:4 NASB).

I used to be what you might call an "emotional" person. I frequently suffered from "hurt feelings," and I lived my daily life playing the "victim." It took some time for me to realize that I could acknowledge those feelings without having to act upon them. I have also learned that emotional intelligence is a rare commodity. However, basic awareness of how our own emotions affect our actions is a must. We have two choices regarding our emotions: They control us, or we control them. Simply reacting upon what we feel causes our critical thinking to be impaired and we lack discernment. This is our emotion controlling us. If we stop to think before we respond, God's wisdom can flow, and we have clear judgment. This is us controlling our emotion. All humans have feelings, but not all feelings should guide our daily life.

Refusing to adapt will only lead to unfruitful struggles.

There was a man who traveled to a big city for the first time. He was so excited that, upon arrival, he found the tallest hotel in town and got himself a room on the upper floor for the night. Once in the room, he pulled open the curtains and looked through the window from on high. As he gazed at the vast view of the city, he noticed that it appeared as though the building was swaying. The more he looked, the more confident he was that the building was actually moving. He immediately called down to the front desk to voice his concern. The clerk on the other end responded by confirming to him that the hotel was indeed swaying and went on to explain that it was doing so out of necessity. It had been designed and built that way in order to withstand the wind, weather, or a possible earthquake. The clerk then offered to gladly move the gentleman to a lower floor if he so desired to. With this new-found revelation, the man was now perfectly comfortable right where he was. That building needed to be flexible in order to endure; being too rigid would cause it to tumble if a powerful storm came. Similarly, being too resistant to accept God's way over ours only impairs our ability to withstand the storms of life. We must be flexible to His will. Going with the flow has its place but sometimes we need to plan ahead as best we can. When my husband and I traveled to Europe last year, I neglected to pack a power adapter for my charger. The outlets there run on a totally different system. Without a European adapter, none of our electronic devices could even be plugged in. It was most inconvenient and caused a serious hiccup in our travel plans. The lack of an adapter made our efforts to charge our electronics futile. Similarly, we will not succeed in surrendering to God if we don't adapt to change. Refusal to adapt is rebellion and will only lead to unfruitful struggles.

John the Baptist set a great example of how to adapt. As a preacher, his message of repentance taught people to change the way they thought and acted. He had many followers who would flock to see him in the wilderness to hear him speak and be baptized. Jesus was no exception. When John was told of the many followers that Jesus had, he said, "He must become greater and greater, and I must become less and less" (John 3:30 NLT). He knew that change had come, and He was willing to give up the life He knew for something much greater to be fulfilled. It was His loyalty to God that enabled Him to do so. Our own loyalty to God will be tested as well, as we travel along the journey of surrender. We will see both immediate and gradual change. We should respond to those changes that mark our success. Proverbs 4:18 tells us, "The path of the righteous is like the morning sun, shining ever brighter till the full light of day." We aren't enlightened all at once; it is a lifelong process. The key is to not only expect change but to *want* change. That is what keeps us on the path of progression. It helps to remind ourselves of how far we have already come and how God has helped us through it all. Psalm 18:16-19 says:

> *He reached down from on high and took*
> *hold of me; he drew me out of deep waters.*
> *He rescued me from my powerful enemy,*

from my foes, who were too strong for me. They confronted me in the day of my disaster, but the Lord was my support. He brought me out into a spacious place; he rescued me because he delighted in me.

Accepting the many changes that our new life in Christ brings can be challenging. But to me, it is just as much adventurous. Just as there are so many exciting things to see in nature when the seasons change, so it is with us as we progress through our many spiritual seasons. Remember there is a time for all things.

In the words of King Solomon:

There is a time for everything,
and a season for every activity under the
heavens:
a time to be born and a time to die,
a time to plant and a time to uproot,
a time to kill and a time to heal,
a time to tear down and a time to build,
a time to weep and a time to laugh,
a time to mourn and a time to dance,
a time to scatter stones and a time to gather
them,
a time to embrace and a time to refrain from
embracing,
a time to search and a time to give up,
a time to keep and a time to throw away,
a time to tear and a time to mend,
a time to be silent and a time to speak,
a time to love and a time to hate,
a time for war and a time for peace.

-Ecclesiastes 3:1-8

HIT ME WITH YOUR BEST SHOT

Nehemiah was assigned with the task of rebuilding the walls of Jerusalem. His enemies were seeking to stop the work, so they sent letters to him asking if he would meet with them: "But they were scheming to harm me; so, I sent messengers to them with this reply: 'I am carrying on a great project and cannot go down. Why should the work stop while I leave it and go down to you?' Four times they sent me the same message, and each time I gave them the same answer" (Nehemiah 6:2-4). A fifth letter was sent that accused him of plotting a revolt and said they were going to report him to the king. Nehemiah replied, "Nothing like what you are saying is happening; you are just making it up out of your head" (Nehemiah 6:8). He knew that they were trying to frighten him and his workers, thinking, "Their hands will get too weak for the work, and it will not be completed" (Nehemiah 6:9). Nehemiah stayed his course and completed the restoring of the wall in fifty-two days. His determination to finish what God had instructed was greater than the persistent approaches of his enemy.

We, too, have an enemy who wants nothing more than for us to "abandon ship" when the seas get rough. *Fear* is a powerful weapon used by our enemy to convince us to back down from our decision to surrender to God. Peter provides a prime example of what can happen when we allow fear to distract us. Peter was with his fellow disciples out on a boat in the middle of a windstorm. He saw Jesus walking on the water and wanted to go to Him. When Jesus beckoned him to come, Peter stepped out of the boat and began walking on the water. As he made his way towards Jesus, he was distracted by the powerful wind, and he took his eyes off Jesus. At that moment, his fear caused him to sink. In much the same way, our faith can be sidelined if we pay attention to fear. James 4:7 tells us to "Resist the devil and he will flee from you." Faith is the opposite of fear, so remain faithfully focused on God to prevent falling prey to fear.

Have you ever done something that you really felt good about, only to see that no one else was impressed? Have you ever been eating right and exercising, only to not lose a single pound? *Discouragement* is one of the most debilitating feelings a person can have, and there seems to be an endless supply of discouraging moments in life. And it doesn't matter who you are. During the Civil War, General Robert E. Lee had a shortage of soldiers. In order to prevent the Union army from finding out and attempting to overthrow his men, he decided to make his Confederate army appear larger than it actually was. He had the same troop of Confederate soldiers loaded onto trains and transported them to various stations, making it seem as though new soldiers were being added to the Rebel army. Those reports confused the Union forces into believing that the enemy was much bigger than it really was. His tactic worked. Similarly, our enemy tries to discourage us by making our struggles seem bigger than they are, but this, too, is just an illusion. We cannot believe everything we see.

I used to enjoy watching Dale Earnhardt, Sr. race. His nickname, "The Intimidator," was earned by his aggressive racing style. No driver appreciated being in front of him. They knew if they saw that black #3 closing in from behind, they would have to move over, or he would do it for them. Many times, his presence was so intimidating that the driver in front of him would crash. Most often, Earnhardt would push his way right through and, on one particular occasion was asked about it after the race. He responded with these words, "I didn't mean to wreck him; I was just trying to rattle his cage."[3] The same strategy was used thousands of years ago by the Philistine army as they taunted the Israelites in the Valley of Elah. Goliath's presence was so forceful that, "On hearing the Philistine's words, Saul and all the Israelites were dismayed and terrified...Whenever the Israelites saw the man, they all fled from him in great fear"(1 Samuel 17:11,24). Goliath was the "intimidator," but David's response was extraordinary:

> *David said to the Philistine, 'You come against me with sword and spear and javelin, but I come against you in the name of the Lord Almighty, the God of the armies of Israel, whom you have defied. This day the Lord will deliver you into my hands, and I'll strike you down and cut off your head. This very day I will give the carcasses of the Philistine army to the birds and the wild animals, and the whole world will know that there is a God in Israel. All those gathered here will know that it is not by sword or spear that the Lord saves; for the battle is the Lord's, and he will give all of you into our hand.'" (1 Samuel 17:45-47)*

Like the Israelite army, feeding into *intimidation* can cause us to lose hope. And when hope is lost, our ability to live boldly is diminished. That is a dangerous place to be. Proverbs 13:12 says that when hope is crushed, so is the heart. With a crushed heart, a man simply cannot act in faith. What has helped me to remain hopeful and encouraged despite circumstance, is dwelling on the truth of God's word, much the way that David did. If God has said it, it is true. Charles Spurgeon is quoted as saying, "A Bible that is falling apart is usually owned by someone who isn't."[4] The more of His word we can allow to penetrate our heart, the bolder the faith we will have to face any enemy. Accepting discouragement and being intimidated is a choice I don't need to make.

We can sometimes unintentionally cause our own failures because of the words we speak. A study was done on how words affect our actions. Researchers placed a small group of preschoolers at a table and gave them all a picture to color. Then they passed out a glass of milk to each child, telling each one not to spill the milk. Nearly all of them ended up spilling the milk. Then, they placed another small group of preschoolers at the same table to color a picture and gave them all a glass of milk. But this time, they told them to keep the milk in the glass. They did. What we hear impresses an image in our subconscious mind, upon which we act. The second direction was posed in a positive way. We see the same strategy used in classrooms. Teachers post rules in a positive fashion. For example, instead of "Don't talk while the teacher is talking" the rule reads "Be quiet while the teacher is talking." Instead of "Don't run in the hallway," the rule is stated as "Always walk in the hallway." We should strive to impress positive images in our mind by speaking positive words. Doing so will inevitably cause us to respond accordingly. During a presentation on the importance of non-violent communication, a billboard was placed at the front of the room filled with the following lines:

WORDSWORDSWORDSWORDSWORDSWORDS
WORDSWORDSWORDSWORDSWORDSWORDS
WORDSWORDSWORDSWORDSWORDSWORDS
WORDSWORDSWORDSWORDSWORDSWORDS
WORDSWORDSWORDSWORDSWORDSWORDS

If you look closely, *words* begin to look like *swords.* What a powerful visual impact! Words can easily become swords if they aren't chosen carefully. Neglecting to pay attention to what we say cannot only hurt others but ourselves as well. Words can be walls or windows. They either imprison us or set us free. No one functions optimally behind bars, so speaking words of freedom are a far better choice. Negativity provides fuel for our enemy and let's face it, he needs no help from us! Positivity is a protection for us: spiritually, emotionally, and physically. The Bible says that out of the heart, the mouth speaks. So, fill your heart with the truth of God's words, be filled with positive images of hope and in due time we will be like those the book of Luke refers to: "having heard the word, [they] keep it, and bring forth fruit with patience" (Luke 8:15 KJV).

Chapter 9

OPERATION: CARRY-ON

I planned ahead and had my boarding pass in hand, but I still had to check my bag in. I took a deep breath as I watched my suitcase travel the conveyor belt into the abyss of the airport's belly, silently wondering if it would make it to "the other side." At my destination, I got off the plane and began the search. I found the right carousel and started weeding through the mob of hovering passengers, who were also anxiously waiting for their bags. One by one, bags appeared and were paired up with their owners. "Where is mine?" I asked myself. Finally, I could see it from a distance and started to make my way, trying to time it just right so as not to miss "the catch." A sigh of relief and a match made in heaven, but then I had to lug it around an unknown airport as I tried to find the exit. *So that's why it's called luggage*, I think to myself. I was soon wishing I had packed much lighter. All my perfect outfits and those "just in case" items were just not necessary. Realistically speaking, I wasn't traveling anywhere that wouldn't have a store nearby if I needed anything. I learned that less is definitely more and that it's so much easier to simply pack a carry-on. I had just made things harder for myself. My luggage story helps to illustrate this concept:

Life itself is a journey and has plenty of opportunity for stressful moments. So, the less you "pack," the less problematic your life will be.

Confucius said, "Life is really simple, but we insist on making it complicated." One of the best ways to make things easier for ourselves is *"possibility* thinking." My over-preparedness in packing only kept me from seeing the opportunity to manage my trip more effectively. Insisting on our own way obscures possibility thinking and without possibility, we can get stuck. Jim Rohn, author and motivational speaker, said that "what is easy to do is also easy not to do."[1] It is very easy to stop and ask for directions. Yet, we would rather waste time driving around in circles because we fail to see the invitation to find out where we need to go, from someone who really knows. We refuse to see the possibility that there is a better way. We must also be aware of our own contributions to our complicated lives.

Simplicity is a word that gets tossed around quite a bit when it comes to lifestyle. But the simple life is different for everyone. There are, however, some universal actions that can be taken to simplify your life.

Know what is most important to you because knowledge is power. Without a clear vision of your priorities, you will inevitably neglect them. Write them down if you need to. How much of what you do is devoted to the things that are most important to you? Be sure you are completely honest with yourself. Sometimes, we can be very busy, yet we're miserable, because we are doing the wrong things. Pay attention to how you spend your time. Tracking it in a journal for a week or so may even help. It could be chores, hobbies, TV, the internet, eating, driving, shopping, even friends or social events. Objectively ask yourself, *how important are those things that I'm spending my time on?* I have heard that knowledge is accumulation, but wisdom is elimination, and I would have to agree. Use your new-found knowledge to make you wiser. Start eliminating, or at least minimizing, the least important things that occupy your life. Those things may quite possibly be taking away from your ability to live comfortably. Personally, I have found that TV watching and social media usage are what I call "time suckers." Time just seems to melt away during those activities. I have also found that even having the option of watching a certain program or checking the latest status update was a mental distraction that took time in thought. So simply put, I quit them both. I now fill my time more wisely with reading, writing, baking, DIY projects, or even meditating.

SIMPLE IS AS SIMPLE DOES

Shortening your to-do list can help, too. Be realistic with what you can do. Don't spread yourself too thin. There is only one you, and your account is with your creator, not the world. Juggling is a skill best left to see performed by circus clowns. When your list of tasks at hand is minimized, you can appreciate what you must do, and you will inevitably be better at what you accomplish. Managing your time is also important, but it is a study in and of itself and styles vary per individual. So, regarding the proper management of time, I will only suggest this one thing. First and foremost, thank God for the time He has given you. Ask Him to guide you in the best use of your time because he does answer prayers. It has truly surprised me what can be achieved in a single day when I give my time to Him first.

Daily life is full of decisions, both large and small. Mark Zuckerberg, the founder of Facebook, once said that deciding what to wear and what to eat each morning are "silly" decisions that waste time. So, every day, he wears his infamous gray t-shirt, pants, and Nikes. When it's cooler, he throws on a blue hoodie. He also eats the same breakfast each day. Simplicity. He says it frees him up to focus on what matters the most to him.[2] I'm not saying that we should throw out our wardrobe or eat only oatmeal every morning, but we should be alert as to what may be distracting us personally and remove it. Vanity was a distraction for me. Every morning I used to put on my make-up and curl my hair. I had the whole caboodle: liners, lipsticks, and shadows in every color, a lash curler, three different hot irons, spritz and sprays of all kinds. Although I still enjoy that on occasion, my daily ritual has changed. I am happy to walk out of the house each day for work with a clean look of freshly brushed hair and a little lip-balm. Not only have I learned to appreciate being natural, but my wallet thanks me, too.

Jesus alluded to the concept of simplicity in His famous Sermon on the Mount:

> *And why do you worry about clothes? See how the flowers of the field grow. They do not labor or spin. Yet I tell you that not even Solomon in all his splendor was dressed like one of these. If that is how God clothes the grass of the field, which is here today and tomorrow is thrown into the fire, will he not much more clothe you—you of little faith? So do not worry, saying, 'What shall we eat?' or 'What shall we drink?' or 'What shall we wear?' For the pagans run after all these things, and your heavenly Father knows that you need them. (Matthew 6:28-32)*

Another key component of simplifying is minimizing your "stuff." It is far better to have six books on a shelf that you read than fifty that just collect dust. It is good to take inventory regularly, to see what you use and what you don't. No one likes to be ignored, so nothing you own should be either. If you haven't used it in some time, let someone else have a go with it. That rainy day you've been waiting for may never come. Mother Theresa said, "The more you have, the more occupied you are. The less you have, the more free you are."[3] De-cluttering and organizing your home and workspace not only gives you peace of mind but saves time, too. Have a place for everything and everything in its place means you don't waste time looking for something that's lost in the chaos. Too much "stuff" lying around is distracting and will prevent you from being able to focus on what's most important. We all have heard that "You are what you eat," but you are also what you see, feel, hear and smell. Living in a disorderly, cramped, noisy, or dirty environment has a negative effect on your ability to have clarity. Conversely, a clean, organized, calming environment helps to promote a clear positive outlook.

In order to be content in life, we may have to be willing to give some things up. If God has brought us to a place of peace, our lives should reflect that.

In Matthew 6:22-23 Jesus said, "The eye is the lamp of the body; so then if your eye is *clear*, your whole body will be full of light. But if your eye is bad, your whole body will be full of darkness. If then the light that is in you is darkness, how great is the darkness!" The Greek word for *clear* literally means "without folds." That may seem odd to us today, but in that day, it would have made perfect sense. The holy writings were written on scrolls of papyrus that would have to be rolled out in order to be read by lamplight. The primitive lighting, alone, would have made reading and writing a challenge. But if the papyrus had a "fold" in it—a common-day crease—it would be even more difficult to read. Jesus was saying that it is not so much the condition of our eyes that hinders our sight, but what we place in front of them. Distractions can become "folds" in our lives that cause us to lose focus.

One of the simplest joys I have is to be able to enjoy the things I have worked hard to get. King Solomon said that we should enjoy the fruits of our labor, for they are gifts from God (Ecclesiastes 3:13). Hoarding things that will never be used is simply irrational. Jesus reminds us, "Don't store up treasures here on earth, where moths eat them and rust destroys them, and where thieves break in and steal. Store your treasures in heaven, where moths and rust cannot destroy, and thieves do not break in and steal. Wherever your treasure is, there the desires of your heart will also be" (Matthew 6:19-21 NLT). In order to be content in life, we may have to be willing to give some things up. If God has brought us to a place of peace, our lives should reflect that.

THAT'S WHAT I THOUGHT

Simplicity in our thought life is also important. Einstein said that the most important decision we make is to believe we live in either a friendly or hostile environment. I don't know that it is the most important decision, but it does have its relevancy. Choosing the right environment does determine our behavior. I choose to believe as Paul did, that the power of Jesus Christ remains over me like a tent (2 Corinthians 12:9). Regardless of the circumstances in my life, Christ alone is my refuge. Because belief causes action, choosing what to believe is of utmost importance. Figuring out what to fill our minds and hearts with can be challenging and time-consuming. I figured out that building my belief system on the truth of God's word manifests stability, integrity, and peace in my life. Trying to weed through the abundance of "could be" or "should be" truths of the world complicates my life.

One of the infamous scenes from the O.J. Simpson trial of 1995 occurred when O.J. was ordered to try on the gloves that were presented as evidence from the prosecutor's office. The gloves did not fit. Johnny Cochran, O.J.'s attorney, used the following statement in his closing argument to the jury: "If it doesn't fit, you must acquit."[4] Regardless of how you or I may feel about that trial or his guilt or innocence, that statement was inarguable, and it led to O.J.'s acquittal. I use the very same statement to monitor any thought that I have or words that I hear. I filter all of them through God's word, and *if it does not fit* in it, then I *must acquit* it. This simple strategy has had the single biggest impact on my thought life. It is yet another example of how God's plan is best for us. If we trust ourselves to His hands, we can't go wrong.

There was a father who would frequently take his young son on a walk through their hometown. They made it a habit to stop by the hardware store where on the counter perched a large glass jar full of colorful candies. The owner would tell the little boy to go ahead a get some candy, but the boy never reached into the jar to get any. So, the owner would reach into the jar himself, grab some candy and give it to the little boy. This went on for quite some time and, eventually, the boy's father asked his son why he wouldn't get the candy himself. The little boy said, "Well, my hands are small, but the owner's hands are big. If I let him get the candy for me, I get more." The father was tickled by the boy's wisdom. We can learn a great lesson from this little boy. There are many things in our life that are best left for our heavenly Father to handle. Trying to figure out how to solve problems on our own can complicate our mind and disrupt our peace.

I'VE GOT FRIENDS IN LOW PLACES

For me, one of the most difficult things to simplify was my social life. For as long as I can remember, I have always had a bunch of "friends." I used to spend quite a bit of time with other people, listening to entirely too many "voices." I realized that it was keeping me from discovering who I was in Christ, so I disconnected from them. I even gave up my cell phone, and my husband and I now share one. It has been very liberating. To be clear, I am not saying that having friends is wrong or that friends are a distraction. However, not all friends are beneficial to you. Paul told the Corinthians, "Everything is permissible, but not everything is helpful. Everything is permissible, but not everything builds up" (1 Corinthians 10:23 ISV). One true spiritual friend holds greater value than that of five worldly ones. Unfortunately, though many people may have good intentions, even the best of intentions can be misguided. We must be careful who we spend time with and whose voices are beckoning for our attention. King Solomon said, "Walk with the wise and become wise; associate with fools and get in trouble" (Proverbs 13:20 NLT).

YOU CAN DO IT

Eliminating all the excessive things in your life can be a slow process, but it is worth the effort. Though it may be difficult to give up certain things, you will soon realize how great it feels to be free from them. There were things in my life that, at one point, I never would have thought I could live without. In all honesty, those things were adding more want to my life than contentment. The minimalist approach to life is much easier to handle than trying to deal with too many things. I also keep in mind what is stated in Philippians 4:19, that God supplies all my needs "according to *His* glorious riches in Christ Jesus(BSB). God's omnipotence and omnipresence always sees to it that I am well taken care of. I have come to know the secret Paul spoke of in Philippians:

> *"I am not saying this because I am in need, for I have learned to be content whatever the circumstances. I know what it is to be in need, and I know what it is to have plenty. I have learned the secret of being content in any and every situation, whether well fed or hungry, whether living in plenty or in want. I can do all this through him who gives me strength." (Philippians 4:11-13)*

Living up in the mountains, I see quite a few bears. It makes me think of Baloo from Disney's movie, "The Jungle Book." His most famous song includes these lyrics: *"It's the bare necessities, the simple bare necessities. Forget about your worries and your strife. I mean the bare necessities. That's why a bear can rest at ease, with just the bare necessities of life."* He instructs Mowgli, the man-cub: *"Don't spend your time lookin' around for something you want that can't be found. When you find out you can live without it and go along not thinkin' about it. I'll tell you something true, the bare necessities of life will come to you."* [5]

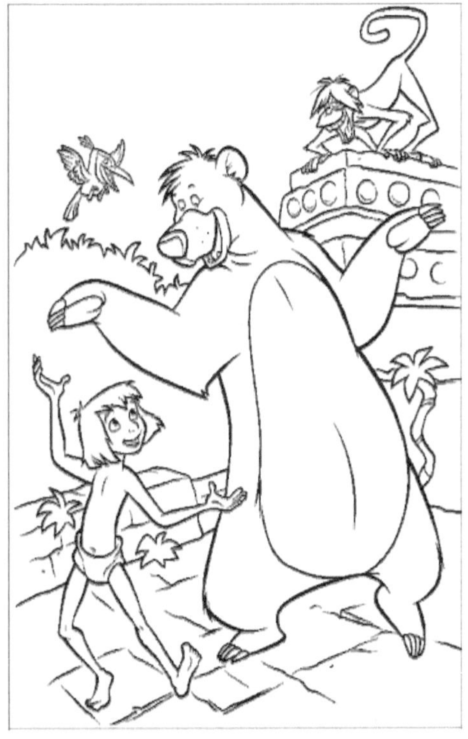

©DISNEY

It's a lighthearted way of teaching such a deep truth. Baloo's lesson reminds us that choosing to focus our time on spiritual things enables us to live peacefully with our needs simply met. Scripture tells us, "But seek first the kingdom of God and His righteousness, and all these things will be added unto you" (Matthew 6:33 BSB). We are reminded that God is in control. We are to rest easy in that knowledge. Although living care-free in the jungle may sound exciting, real life often presents challenges that cannot be cured by a simple song and dance.

In those cases, perseverance is necessary to keep it simple. The word persevere is the combination of two Greek words meaning "to remain" and "to be under." Remaining under God's protection, guidance, grace, and love is really the key to the simple life. Jesus mastered that, although most people would look at the life of Jesus and say that it was far from a simple one. I would have to disagree. His responsibility was great, yes. His task at hand was difficult, yes. But simple doesn't mean you have no obligation or that life is a piece of cake. It means that you have a clear vision and oversight beyond condition. Jesus relied on God's strength and direction throughout His life, death, and ultimate resurrection. Moments before His arrest in the garden of Gethsemane He prayed, "Yet not as I will, but as You will" (Matthew 26:39). Christopher Reeve, aka Superman, said that "A hero is an ordinary individual who finds the strength to persevere and endure in spite of overwhelming obstacles."[6] Notice that he said finding the strength not having the strength. Often, there is a small part of us all that would love to be the superhero of our own life, but it is much more important to have God's supernatural intervention instead. It is in acknowledging that it is not within our own strength, but in finding God's strength, that we can succeed. Once we open the doors to the wealth of God's power in our lives, we open a world of possibilities. We become free to live the lives we were intended to live, the life that Jesus spoke of in this passage from Matthew:

"Therefore, I tell you, do not worry about your life, what you will eat or drink; or about your body, what you will wear. Is not life more than food, and the body more than clothes? Look at the birds of the air; they do not sow or reap or store away in barns, and yet your heavenly Father feeds them. Are you not much more valuable than they? Can any one of you by worrying add a single hour to your life?" (Matthew 6:25-27)

Our Heavenly Father knows what you need, when you need it. The only thing you are required to do is seek Him and rest in the simple truth of this statement: God loves you. And that is really all you need to know.

THE HEART OF THE MATTER

You, your life, your light. That is the real heart of the matter. Mankind spends countless hours—even years—seeking significance in the world, only to find none. To me, that is the greatest travesty of life. I am not saying that our pursuit of happiness is superficial or that our desire to "be somebody" is a farce. Those are both human needs. I just don't believe we are taught to look for those things in the right place. The whole human race spends entirely too much time looking outward rather than inward, comparing ourselves to one another, just trying to belong. Popular competitive reality shows, like American Idol and The Apprentice, dictate to us that our value is based on performing better than everyone else—all while subjecting ourselves to the scrutiny of fellow human beings. To what gain? According to published data, twenty percent of Americans experience some type of mental illness during their lifetime. Millions of dollars are being poured into our economy on cosmetic surgery and self-improvement programs. More and more people are attempting to "find themselves" by recreating or altering their identity. Society's perverse values and lack of Biblical standards have affected us all. We endure the injustice— the "slings and arrows"—of this world, and we become angry or disappointed. Even the best of us are prey to failure, shame, and confusion. Happiness and contentment seem to elude mankind.

The human condition of imperfection is universal. Romans tells us that "There is no distinction, for all have sinned and fall short of the glory of God and are justified freely by His grace" (Romans 3:22-24 BSB). Regardless of where we have been or what we have done in life, our Creator meets us right where we are. We needn't explain anything to Him because He already knows it all. Hebrews 4:13 says that "Everything is uncovered and laid bare before the eyes of him to whom we must give account." God loves us and wants to work through us, flaws and all. Noah got drunk. Abraham lied. Moses was a murderer. Rahab was a harlot. David was an adulterer. Jonah ran away. Peter denied Christ. God can work with those character flaws, with people who have a rocky past or even a questionable present. What we perceive as a flaw may very well be used by God for our splendor and His ultimate glory.

There exists the living and loving God who has already gifted within us all we need to prosper and live fulfilled. Each one of us is unique and designed with divine purpose. We have the definitive presence of God within us and all around us. Believe it. Benjamin Franklin said, "There are three things that are extremely hard: Steel, diamonds and to know one's own self." However, I believe it is only difficult to know ourselves when we are trying to be someone we were not created to be. The Gospel of Thomas reads in verse three, "When you come to know yourself, then you will become known and you will realize that it is you who are the sons of the living Father. But if you will not know yourself, you dwell in poverty and it is you who are that poverty." Poverty is simply the state of being inferior in quality or insufficient in amount. Without spiritual enlightenment of who we truly are, we live impoverished. God has placed a rich existence within the hearts of all men, for this life and for eternity. That is a priceless gift and can only be discovered in Jesus Christ, for man's efforts cannot satisfy that hidden desire. We look into mirrors every day to see our natural reflection but peering into Christ reveals our divine self. Paul said it this way,

"For now we see in a mirror dimly, but then face to face; now I know in part, but then I will know fully just as I also have been fully known"(1 Corinthians 13:12 NASB). True and ultimate satisfaction is found only at the very core of who we were created to be.

***But now, O Lord, You are our Father;
we are the clay, and You the potter;
and we are all the work of Your hand.
(Isaiah 64:8 BSB)***

It is impossible for any of us to be faultless, to know all things or to have everything we want. But God is fair and just. Trust him. Learning to do so and to allow His ways to operate ours is the greatest gift we can give ourselves and the world. 2 Corinthians 3:3 says, "You show that you are a letter of Christ... written not with ink but with the Spirit of the living God, not on tablets of stone but on tablets of human hearts." It is a *privilege* and an *honor* to have the light of Christ reflected in our lives. He promises to transform us from glory to glory when we surrender to Him. Ask not what it will cost you, but what it will cost if you don't. Being humbled under the mighty hand of God leads to being exalted in due time, for all who have given up all will be given more. Jesus said, "I have told you these things, so that in me you may have peace. In this world you will have trouble. But take heart! I have overcome the world" (John 16:33).

There may be no "easy" button for life, but faith does work miracles. Cast all your burdens on God because He cares for you. Hanging on to them will only get in the way of the life God has planned for you. Psalm 37:3-6 says to:

"Trust in the Lord and do good; dwell in the land and enjoy safe pasture. Take delight in the Lord, and he will give you the desires of your heart. Commit your way to the Lord trust in him and he will do this: He will make your righteous reward shine like the dawn, your vindication like the noonday sun."

As the potter, God continues to lovingly mold me day by day. As the clay in His hands, I can say with conviction that he is truly making a masterpiece of my life.

I waited patiently for the Lord to help me,
and he turned to me and heard my cry.
He lifted me out of the pit of despair,
out of the mud and the mire.
He set my feet on solid ground
and steadied me as I walked along.
He has given me a new song to sing,
a hymn of praise to our God.
Many will see what he has done and be amazed.
They will put their trust in the Lord.
Oh, the joys of those who trust the Lord,
who have no confidence in the proud
or in those who worship idols.
O Lord my God, you have performed
many wonders for us.
Your plans for us are too numerous to list.
You have no equal.
If I tried to recite all your wonderful deeds,
I would never come to the end of them.
(Psalm 40:1-5 NLT)

To him be the glory forever and ever. Amen.

JUST FOR YOUR OWN THOUGHTS...

NOTES

Chapter 1 : Playing Possum
1. Denzel Washington, https://speakola.com/grad/denzel-washington-everything-i-have-is-by-the-grace-of-god-full-2015
2. Hans Christian Andersen, *The Ugly Duckling*, 1843
3. Myles Munroe, https://en.wikipedia.org/wiki/Myles_Munroe
4. *The Little Mermaid*, Walt Disney Pictures, 1989
5. Joni Eareckson Tada, https://en.wikipedia.org/wiki/Joni_Eareckson_Tada
6. Alexander Pope, https://en.wikipedia.org/wiki/Alexander_Pope

Chapter 2 : Ditch the Floaties
1. Alexander Pope, https://www.azquotes.com/author/11775-Alexander_Pope
2. Honest John, *Pinocchio*, Walt Disney Pictures, 1940
3. Microsoft, https://medicalxpress.com/news/2015-05-microsoft-human-attention-span-lags.html
4. Yogi Berra, https://bible.org/illustration/yogi-berra-0
5. Gyalwang Karmapa, https://news.harvard.edu/gazette/story/2015/03/the-most-dangerous-thing-in-the-world-is-apathy/
6. Pink Floyd, *Comfortably Numb*, The Wall, 1979
7. Martin Luther King, https://www.goodreads.com/quotes/16312-faith-is-taking-the-first-step-even-when-you-can-t

Chapter 3 : Let's Talk About Love
1. Andre Gide, https://www.insightoftheday.com/motivational-quote-by-andre-gide-03-05-2019
2. Lucille Ball, https://www.brainyquote.com/quotes/lucille_ball_127076

Chapter 4 : Can't Touch This – The Grandeur of God
1. Washington Carver, http://thinkexist.com/quotation/i_love_to_think_of_nature_as_an_unlimited/206757.html
2. Gary Starkweather, https://www.andalusiastarnews.com/2016/04/16/some-inventions-were-uniquely-inspired-2/

Chapter 5 : There's Something About Jesus
1. Joseph Scriven, *What a friend we have in Jesus*, https://library.timelesstruths.org/music/What_a_Friend_We_Have_in_Jesus/

2.   John Newton, http://www.cslewisinstitute.org/Amazing_Grace_page5
3.   Bob Marley, *Redemption Song,* Uprising, 1980

Chapter 6 : I Can See Clearly Now
1.   Naval Operations transcript,
      https://en.wikipedia.org/wiki/Lighthouse_and_naval_vessel_urban_
      legend
2.   Author Unknown, *Be careful little eyes*,
      https://library.timelesstruths.org/texts/Treasures_of_the_Kingdom_49/Be
      _Careful_Little_Eyes/

Chapter 7 : How Does Your Garden Grow?
1.   Masaru Emoto, https://www.mynaturalhealer.com/dr-emoto-water-
      experiments/
2.   James Allen, *As a Man Thinketh*, 1903
3.   James Cameron, *Avatar,* Lightstorm Entertainment, 2009
4.   C.S. Lewis, https://www.bloggingtheologically.com/2015/12/11/what-cs-
      lewis-wrote-is-better-than-what-he-didnt/
5.   C.S. Lewis, https://www.goodreads.com/quotes/37169-courage-is-not-
      simply-one-of-the-virtues-but-the
6.   Stephen Crane, *The Red Badge of Courage,* 1895

Chapter 8 : I Never Promised You a Rose Garden
1.   Joe South, *Rose garden*, Introspect, 1968
2.   Woodrow Wilson, https://quotescover.com/woodrow-wilson-quote-
      about-loyalty
3.   Dale Earnhardt, http://thinkexist.com/quotes/dale_earnhardt/
4.   Charles Spurgeon, https://www.goodreads.com/quotes/397346-a-bible-
      that-s-falling-apart-usually-belongs-to-someone-who

Chapter 9 : Operation Carry-on
1.   Jim Rohn, https://quotefancy.com/quote/838207/Jim-Rohn-What-is-easy-
      to-do-is-also-easy-no-to-do
2.   Mark Zuckerberg, https://www.businessinsider.com/barack-obama-mark-
      zuckerberg-wear-the-same-outfit
3.   Mother Theresa, https://www.goodreads.com/quotes/805731-the-more-
      you-have-the-more-you-are-occupied-the
4.   Johnnie Cochran, https://brainyquote.com/quotes/johnnie_
      cochran_191505
5.   Terry Gilkyson, Bare Necessities, The Jungle Book, 1967,
      http://www.songlyrics.com/jungle-book-the-soundtrack/the-bare-
      necessities-lyrics/
6.   Christopher Reeve, https://brainyquote.com/authors/christopher_reeve

All images used are public domain, unless otherwise noted.

Answer:
There's Something About Jesus Word Search

```
W H N P U R N H D X W E X A M P L E N R
D R E H P E H S D O O G H A P M C Y W V
L M D K V G H I G H P R I E S T U C D V
M X D Y S F B R T L T A E N B M E C N X
J J H D K L T J F Y L R F A O B K P N H
R G J L S O N J F K B L I C W I R D H D
S E L E T S N X U V R H S N Y C L Q W P
U G H N X A B S B R E A D O F L I F E I
A L H T H H H K B G O F U T H S I N O Q
W Q N L A B M A L F L A B T I B O U L C
B K N M N F O J A I M R U M K B U B X A
I I E B U N F U H G Y R I L L D C S J F
D V Y A G W H A T S T A X E G D U J F G
L D O M D X Y O Y G R Y A W R H D A Y A
R G J I I K V C A A I B H T T T L U I A
O R F W Y A E T B U F O G S D V H A M J
W R Q P T K D B R A T S G N I N R O M B
E N E D B P I R F T F T W X C I T D H J
H E N D P Q M E O S O X L L T H C D S F
T H E I E U X F N W N A Y T J T A M N V
F F A M B E E I T N E U O C D E T A X Q
O S E V B O M L T M K H P A N R P Q R I
T T W X W W B E C Q R B T M E Q O N G U
H J T Y B C Q P R E L Y B R I O W L A O
G C V L T F F V C V O C M T R N X G G O
I F F P O O R E S M X U J M F S Q M J T
L C M P E X W F N O C J W A U L A Q U X
M G S O M R W H M B I V H D D E T X B H
S J A D C I O X A W M C U N W N I W D L
B P R I N C E O F P E A C E O R L F G C
```

**SON FATHER REDEEMER PRINCEOFPEACE GOODSHEPHERD JUDGE
LION LAMB LORD FRIEND HIGHPRIEST WAY TRUTH LIFE EXAMPLE
LIGHTOFTHEWORLD THEWORD MORNINGSTAR BREADOFLIFE RABBI**

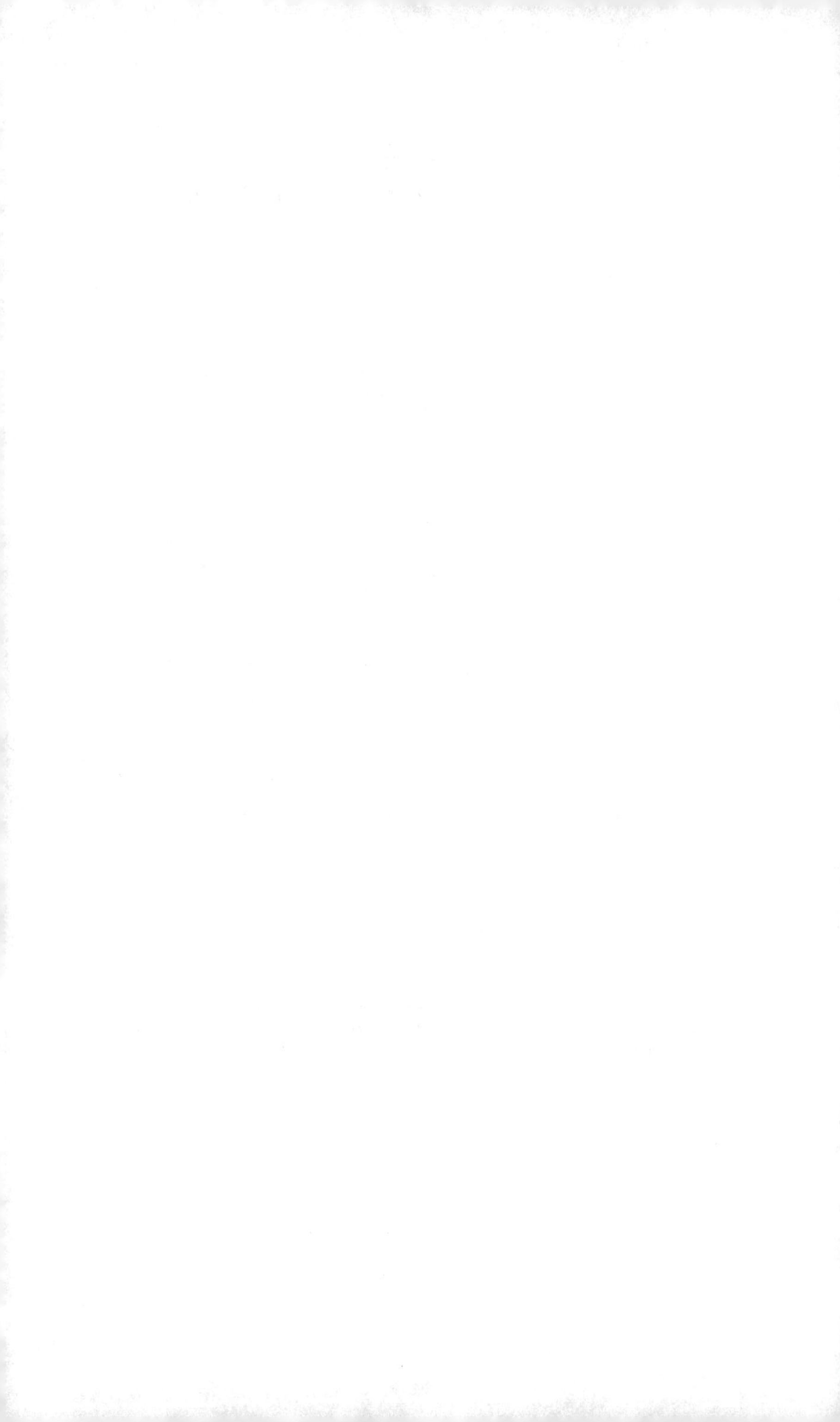